What you gonna do when you get back?
Take a shower and hit the rack.
NO WAY!
PT, PT every day,
Build your body the Academy way.

TRADITIONAL NAVAL ACADEMY CADENCE

"Excellence without arrogance."

AN UNOFFICIAL MOTTO OF THE UNITED STATES NAVAL ACADEMY

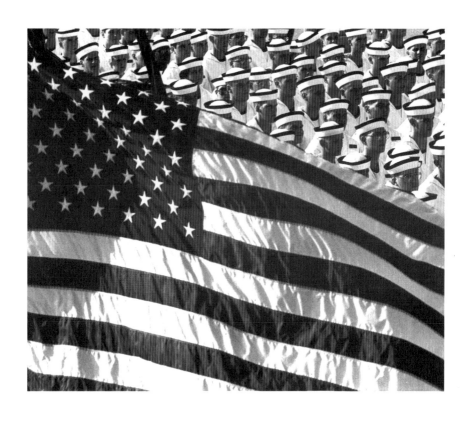

THE OFFICIAL
UNITED STATES
NAVAL ACADEMY
WORKOUT

RESEARCHED BY
ANDREW FLACH

PHOTOGRAPHED BY
PETER FIELD PECK

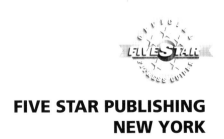

FIVE STAR PUBLISHING
NEW YORK

Five Star Publishing
An Independent Imprint of Hatherleigh Press

Five Star Publishing
1114 First Avenue, Suite 500
New York, NY 10021
1-800-906-1234
www.getfitnow.com

Before beginning any strenuous exercise program consult your physician. The
author and publisher of this book and workout disclaim any liability,
personal or professional, resulting from the misapplication of any of the
training procedures described in this publication.

A portion of the proceeds from the sale of each book will be donated to the
United States Naval Academy Alumni Association.

All Five Star Publishing titles are available for bulk purchase, special
promotions, and premiums. For more information, please contact the manager
of our Special Sales Department at 1-800-906-1234.

Library of Congress Cataloging-in-Publication Data

Flach, Andrew, 1961 –
The official United States Naval Academy workout / researched by Andrew Flach :
photographed by Peter Field Peck
p.   cm. — (Official Five Star fitness guides)
ISBN 1–57826–010–8 (pbk.   alk. paper)
1. Exercise.   2. Physical fitness.   3. United States Naval Acade   I. Title.
II. Series: Flach, Andrew, 1961– Official Five Star fitness guides.
GV481.F552   1998
613.7'1—dc21   98–18120
                                              CIP

Cover design by Gary Szczecina
Text design and composition by DC Designs
Photographed by Peter Field Peck
with Canon® cameras and lenses on·Fuji® print and slide film
except for photos on pages 2, 5, 7, 16, 18-19, 22, 24, 27-29,
courtesy of The U.S. Naval Academy

Printed in the United States of America on acid-free paper
10 9 8 7 6 5 4 3 2 1

MISSION OF THE UNITED STATES NAVAL ACADEMY

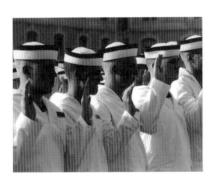

To develop midshipmen morally, mentally and physically and to imbue them with the highest ideals of duty, honor and loyalty in order to provide graduates who are dedicated to a career of naval service and have potential for future development in mind and character to assume the highest responsibilities of command, citizenship and government.

ACKNOWLEDGMENTS

I would like to thank the following individuals and organizations for their time, effort, and support:

United States Naval Academy Public Affairs Office

Special thanks to:
Rear Admiral Thomas Jurowsky
Former Public Affairs Officer, USNA

Elizabeth Kucik
Media Relations Specialist

Karen Myers
Director of Media Relations

Ensign Leslie Hull-Ryde, US Navy

Coach Ed Perry
Deputy Physical Education Officer

Navy Office of Information
Pentagon, Washington, DC

Special thanks to:
Rear Admiral Kendall Pease
Chief of Information

Lieutenant Wendy Snyder
Public Affairs Officer

Our editorial team: Susan Ruszala and Heather Ogilvie
Our design and production team:
Dede Cummings, Matt Sharff, and Gary Szczecina
Our logistics and support team: Kevin Moran and Bruce Slagle
And to the many others who contributed
to the success of this mission: Thank you!

DEDICATION

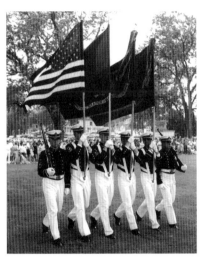

To Heinz Lenz, who for 20 years raised to new levels the standard of physical excellence at the United States Naval Academy. May his efforts inspire midshipmen today and tomorrow.

CONTENTS

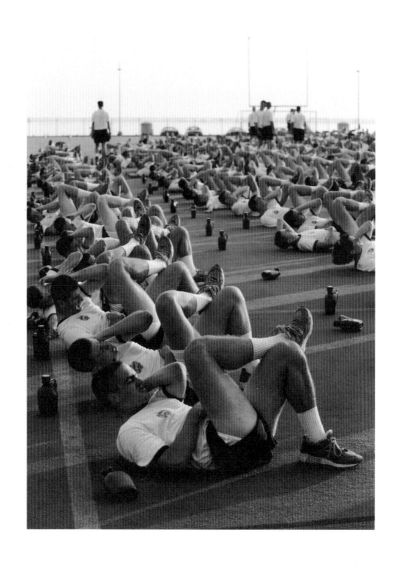

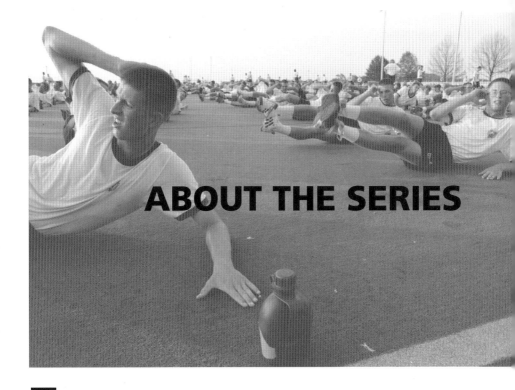

ABOUT THE SERIES

The Five Star Official Fitness Guides are designed to provide a fresh new perspective on the subject of personal health and fitness by documenting the physical training regimens of the United States Armed Forces.

To bring you this exciting information, we have shouldered our gear in the hot midday sun, on cold frosty mornings, in the dark of night. No workouts and training schedules were reorganized to meet our needs. Nor did we ask. We wanted to bring to you what's REAL. I like to think of these books as "fitness documentaries" —because that's what they are!

We have talked extensively with many individuals responsible for the physical fitness and welfare of the men and women of America's Armed Forces. We have discovered the most powerful workout and physical training routines in the world. We bring them to you with the hope that you will be inspired to value your health and pursue fitness activities throughout your life.

Wherever possible, primary source material is utilized. Documentation, interviews, briefs — all were assembled and culled for details and insights.

Important note: These books are not designed to be follow-to-the-letter workouts. That was never our intention. These books are a collection of information on the subject of fitness and physical training in the US military, full of techniques, routines, hints, suggestions, and tips you can learn from. Your workout should be individualized. We highly recommend you review your fitness plan with a certified trainer, coach, or other individual who possesses the proper knowledge to advise you in such a manner. And of course, consult your physician before commencing any new fitness program or before you intensify your current regimen.

Good luck and may lifelong fitness be your goal!

Andrew Flach
Peter Field Peck

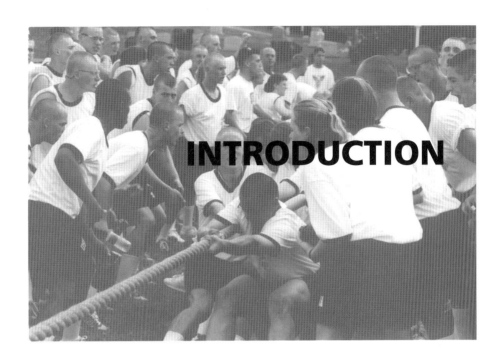

INTRODUCTION

WELCOME ABOARD!

In these pages you'll discover the fitness conditioning secrets of the US Naval Academy. Each summer, more than 1,500 new midshipmen arrive from every corner of the nation. Some are in excellent physical shape and have been successful competitive athletes in high school. Most are of average fitness. And some are below average. Some are tall. Some are short. Some are thin. Some are stocky. Nevertheless they will all go through P.T. together.

The incoming midshipmen, men and women, are known as "plebes" and their first summer of training is known as "plebe summer." Every morning, commencing at 6:00 am sharp, they attend the Physical Education Program, or P.E.P.

P.E.P is conducted on an astroturf field, located in the southeastern area of the USNA campus. Officially known as the Rip Miller Field, more commonly known as the P.E.P. Field, it is the site of intense physical activity on a scale never seen by most people. All 1,500 or so plebes file neatly onto the P.E.P. field to commence their daily P.T. On rainy days, P.E.P takes place in the nearby Halsey Field House.

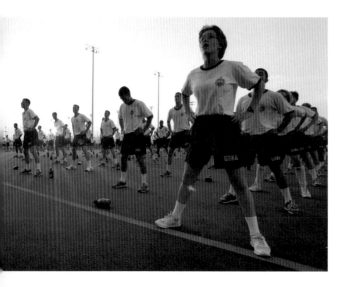

P.E.P. consists of stretching, running, upper body, lower body, and abdominal strengthening exercises coordinated by a team of Company Commanders, Squad Leaders, Platoon Commanders, and Detailers.

This fitness guide documents the P.E.P. of plebe summer 1997. Led by Navy SEALs, the elite Special Forces Unit of the US Navy, 1997's P.E.P. presented a rigorous physical challenge to all incoming midshipmen.

The goal of P.E.P. is simple: to make certain that the men and women of the incoming class are able to successfully pass the US Navy Physical Readiness Test, or PRT. The PRT requirements are as follows:

	Men	*Women*
Pushups	No less than 40	No less than 18
Curl-ups*	No less than 65	No less than 65
Timed 1.5-mile Run	No greater than 10 min. 30 sec.	No greater than 12 min. 38 sec.

* A curl-up is performed as follows: Lie flat on the back; flex knees, thighs 45 degrees to deck, legs shoulder width apart, heels not more than 10 inches from the buttocks, arms folded across chest, hands touching shoulders. Feet flat on the deck are held by a partner only on insteps. From starting position, curl-up until the head is directly above knees. When shoulder blades touch the deck, one repetition has been completed. Do as many repetitions as possible in two minutes.

For individuals who are recovering from P.E.P.-related injuries—quite often shin splints and impact-related injuries—a Water P.E.P. is conducted simultaneously and used as the standard P.E.P. The Water P.E.P. stresses cardio-conditioning, and by being in the water, injuries are not exacerbated. This guide does not cover the Water P.E.P. as it is a remedial program and not the core fitness regimen encountered at plebe summer.

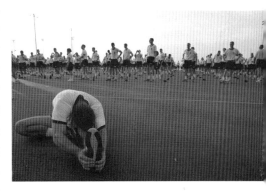

As presented, this guide provides excellent fitness preparatory guidelines for any young man or woman interested in attending the United States Naval Academy, or who has been accepted and is awaiting plebe summer. For those who have not chosen a career as an officer in the United States Navy, it is our hope that this book will distill valuable information and demonstrate proper fitness and conditioning techniques that you can use as a part of your own personal fitness program.

As we've said before, the only caveat is that you consult your physician before commencing any new workout program and that you seek the advice of a qualified fitness professional so you can tailor this workout plan to suit your own personal fitness goals.

Welcome aboard, courtesy of the United States Naval Academy. May health and wellness be your destination.

Andrew Flach

Throughout this book, whenever you see this icon, look for an interesting fact about the Naval Academy that you may not have known. These were taken from *Reef Points*, a manual for incoming plebes. For more information about *Reef Points*, see page 31.

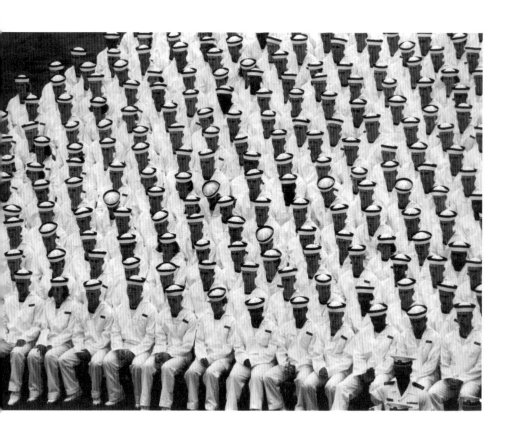

THE UNITED STATES NAVAL ACADEMY TODAY: EXCELLENCE, INTEGRITY, AND TRADITION

THE MISSION

The Naval Academy has a unique clarity of purpose, expressed in its official mission: "To develop midshipmen morally, mentally and physically and to imbue them with the highest ideals of duty, honor and loyalty in order to provide graduates who are dedicated to a career of naval service and have potential for future development in mind and character to assume the highest responsibilities of command, citizenship and government." This puts everyone—faculty, staff and midshipmen—on the same wavelength. It also encourages a sense of spirit and pride found at few other schools.

The moral, mental and physical elements of the USNA program are equally important, all contributing to the qualities of an outstanding naval officer.

ACADEMICS

Every midshipman's academic program begins with a core curriculum that includes courses in engineering, science, mathematics, humani-

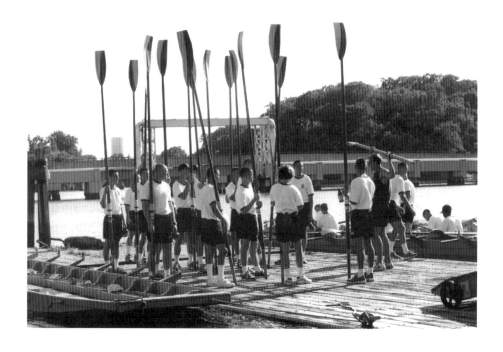

ties and social science. This is designed to give a broad-based education so that a midshipman will qualify for practically any career field in the Navy or Marine Corps. At the same time, the USNA majors program gives midshipmen the opportunity to develop particular areas of academic interest. For especially capable and highly motivated students, the academy offers challenging honors programs and opportunities to start work on postgraduate degrees while still at the Academy.

PROFESSIONAL AND LEADERSHIP TRAINING

After four years at the Naval Academy, the life and customs of naval service become second nature. Midshipmen quickly learn to take orders from practically everyone. But before long, they acquire the responsibility for making decisions that can affect hundreds of other midshipmen. Their professional classroom studies are backed by many hours of practical experience in leadership and naval operations, including assignments with Navy and Marine Corps units during summer months.

MORAL EDUCATION

Moral-ethical development is a fundamental element of all aspects of the Naval Academy experience. As future officers in the Navy or Marine Corps, midshipmen will someday be responsible for the priceless lives of many men and women and multi-million dollar equipment. From plebe summer through graduation, the Naval Academy's four-year character development program focuses on the attributes of integrity, honor, and mutual respect. One of the goals of this program is to develop midshipmen who possess a clear sense of their own moral beliefs and the ability to articulate them. Honor is emphasized by means of the Honor Concept— a system which was originally formulated in 1951 and states, "Midshipmen are persons of integrity: they stand for that which is right." These Academy words to live by are based on the moral values of respect for human dignity, respect for honesty, and respect for the property of others. Brigade honor committees composed of elected

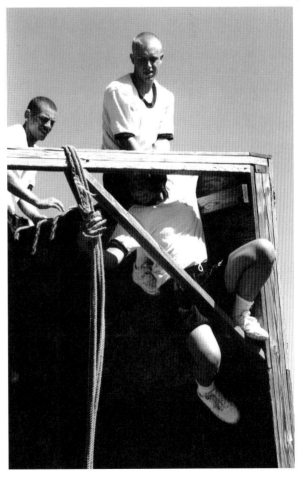

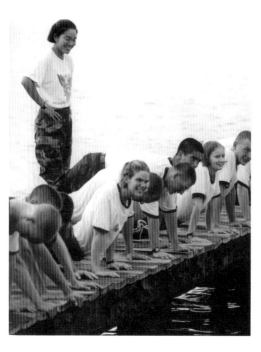

upperclass midshipmen are responsible for education and training in the Honor Concept. Midshipmen found in violation of the Honor Concept by their peers may be separated from the Naval Academy.

THE PHYSICAL MISSION

The mission of the Naval Academy Athletic Department is to develop physical education and athletic programs that exceed fleet standards and foster personal fitness, health, and sportsmanship. These programs prepare Midshipmen for the physical demands of the Navy and instill the interest and knowledge for continued lifetime fitness.

This objective is accomplished through a demanding Physical Education Curriculum and a variety of varsity, club, and intramural sports. Physical education classes are designed to ensure that basic physical mission requirements are met. The primary objectives are:

1. Maximum development of strength, endurance, flexibility, and basic physical skills while stressing the importance of lifetime fitness.

2. Opportunities to develop qualities of physical courage, quick thinking under pressure in highly competitive situations, leadership ability, loyalty, and fair play.

3. Proficiency in aquatics and confidence in meeting emergency conditions in the water.

4. Ability and confidence in defending against personal attack.

5. Interest and expertise in lifetime sports coupled with a fundamental understanding of nutrition, conditioning, and wellness to ensure a continued high level of physical fitness and general well-being following graduation.

These objectives are accomplished through a four-year, 128-hour physical education curriculum. The curriculum includes 40 hours of swimming, 32 hours of personal defense training, 24 hours of physical development training, and 32 hours of recreational sports instruction. Midshipmen fitness levels are also checked once each semester with the same physical readiness test administered in the fleet. This test consists of pushups, curl-ups and a timed 1.5-mile run.

The latitude of Annapolis is 38' 58'.8 North.

The longitude is 76' 29'.3 West.

Varsity, intramural and club sports further contribute to the physical mission by promoting teamwork, leadership, self-confidence, discipline, mental health and the development of lifetime skills.

The Academy emphasizes the importance of being physically fit and prepared for stress because the duties of Navy and Marine Corps officers often require long, strenuous hours in difficult situations. The physical requirements of plebe summer training, four years of physical education, and year-round athletics also develop pride, teamwork and leadership.

THE FUTURE

The classes now at the Naval Academy will produce many of the leaders of the Navy and Marine Corps for the next 30 years. In the course of their careers, the military and political circumstances of the world will take unexpected turns. Military force structures will change as new technology takes hold. Naval Academy graduates will meet these new challenges with courage, honor, and integrity, upholding cherished traditions, always leading to a new and better future.

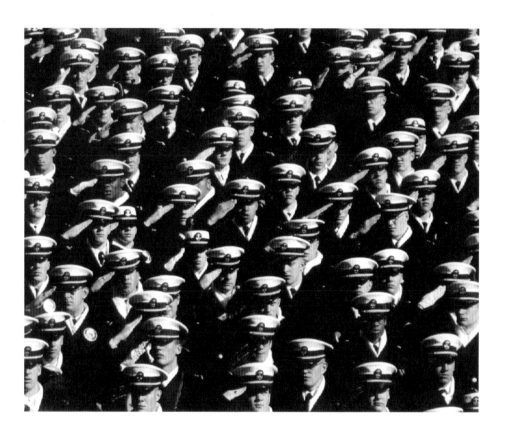

A BRIEF HISTORY OF THE UNITED STATES NAVAL ACADEMY

In 1800, President John Adams made the first recommendation to Congress for the founding of a naval school, but opposition was strong. In 1825, President John Quincy Adams again urged Congress to establish a Naval Academy "for the formation of scientific and accomplished officers." There was a definite need for this school, because until the Naval Academy was established, midshipmen were supposed to be educated by a school master, one of which was aboard every frigate. Needless to say, the quality of education and attendance was poor. But it took until 1842 for the idea of a shore school similar to West Point to be accepted.

On September 13, 1842, the American Brig *Somers* set sail from the Brooklyn Navy Yard on one of the most significant cruises in American naval history. The *Somers* was a school ship for the training of teenage naval apprentice volunteers who would hopefully be inspired to make the Navy a career. However, discipline deteriorated on the *Somers* and it was determined by a court of inquiry aboard ship that Midshipman Philip Spencer and his two chief confederates, Boatswains Mate Samuel Cromwell and Seaman Elisha Small, were guilty of a "determined attempt to commit a mutiny."

The three were hanged at the yardarm and the incident cast doubt over the wisdom of sending midshipmen directly aboard ship to learn

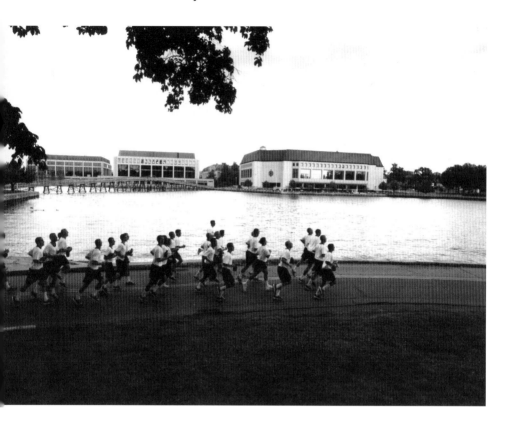

by doing. News of the *Somers* mutiny shocked the country. When Secretary of the Navy Bancroft heard of the hanging of Midshipman Spencer (incidentally the young son of the Secretary of War), he determined that a shore school should replace the school ship. He chose as the site for this school a 10-acre Army post named Fort Severn in Annapolis, Maryland, and on October 10, 1845, with a class of 50 midshipmen and seven professors, the Naval School was born.

The Naval Board of Examiners set the following guidelines for the school:

THE 5 BASIC RESPONSES

1. "Yes, sir/ma'am"
2. "No, sir/ma'am"
3. "No excuse, sir/ma'am"
4. "I'll find out, sir/ma'am"
5. "Aye Aye, sir/ma'am"

1. the age of the first-year naval cadet would be 13 to 15 years

2. a practice frigate and a small steamer would be located at the school for practical instruction

3. the program would be a total of six years, two years of study, followed by three years at sea, followed by a year at school aboard the practice frigate before taking the Lieutenant's exam

4. with the exception of calculus, the course of instruction would be identical to the Military Academy's

5. and lastly, that an Academic Board be established consisting of three persons appointed by the Secretary of the Navy to conduct an annual examination of the Naval Cadets.

The guidelines for today's Naval Academy have changed significantly since the Naval Board of Examiners set down its initial guidelines in 1845:

1. Today's first-year midshipmen must be at least 17 years old (though the average age is 18) and can be no older than 22.

2. Calculus is taught today, and the curriculum as a whole is much more extensive.

3. Today's program is only four years, with midshipmen required to do at least 4 weeks of summer training at sea, and another 4 weeks of additional training (this may be completed in Marine Corps or SEAL training, sailing, or in summer school).

4. While the practice frigate is no longer there, today's midshipmen have approximately 40 training boats, called Yard Patrol boats, at their disposal. These are 115 feet diesel propelled vessels resembling mine sweepers.

5. The Academic Board still exists, though its form has changed to include many more members.

The following years were hard times for both the faculty and the student body, but they persevered and in 1846, Richmond Aulick was ranked first, thus becoming the first "official" graduate of the Naval Academy.

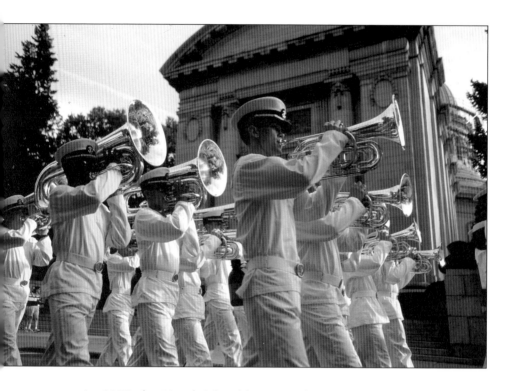

In 1850 the Naval School became the United States Naval Academy. In 1851 a new curriculum went into effect requiring midshipmen to study at the Academy for four years and to train aboard ships each summer. That format is the basis of a far more advanced and sophisticated curriculum at the Naval Academy today.

The *America*, commissioned in 1779 by John Paul Jones, was our first American-built ship of the line.

During the Civil War, the Academy moved temporarily to Fort Adams at Newport, Rhode Island. The first midshipman to resign because of the conflict was W.E. Yancey of Alabama on January 15, 1861.

The year 1873 was an interesting one for the Academy. Albert A. Michelson graduated from the Academy and following a two-year sea tour returned to the Academy where he made his initial experiments on the speed of light. He was the first American to receive a Nobel Prize.

1890 saw the creation of the Navy Athletic Association by Robert Thompson. This was also the year of the first Army-Navy game, which Navy won 20 to 0 on November 29th. By 1891, the Naval Academy Athletic Association was formed under the directorship of Commander Colby Chester. 1892 saw the introduction of the present school colors of blue and gold.

From 1914 through the end of World War I, the size of the Academy's student population increased significantly. In February 1916, the size increased from 1,094 to 1,746.

The Paris Exposition of 1878 presented the Naval Academy with a certificate for "having the best system of education in the United States."

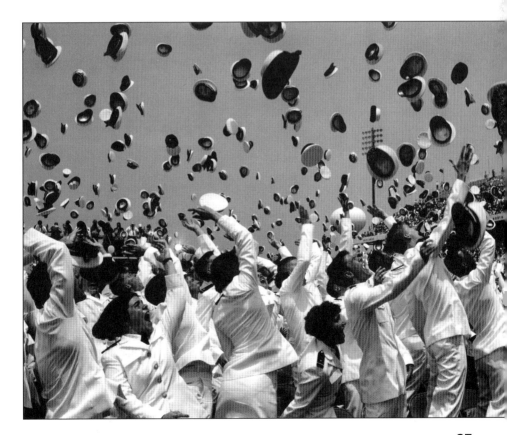

Congress authorized the Naval Academy to begin awarding bachelor of science degrees in 1933. The Academy later replaced a fixed curriculum taken by all midshipmen with the present core curriculum, plus 18 major fields of study, a wide variety of elective courses and

As the US Navy grew over the years, the Academy expanded. The campus of 10 acres increased to 338. The original student body of 50 midshipmen grew to a brigade size of 4,000. Modern granite buildings replaced the old wooden structures of Fort Severn.

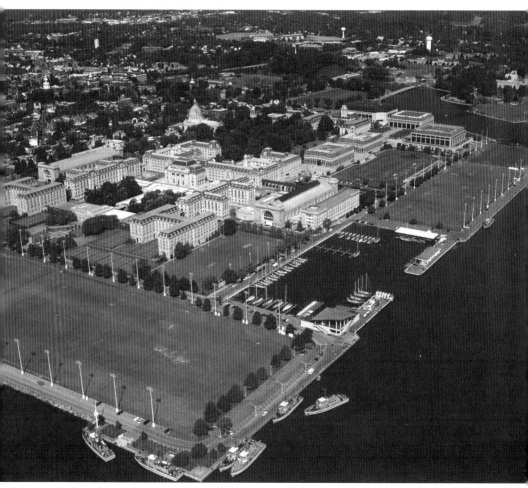

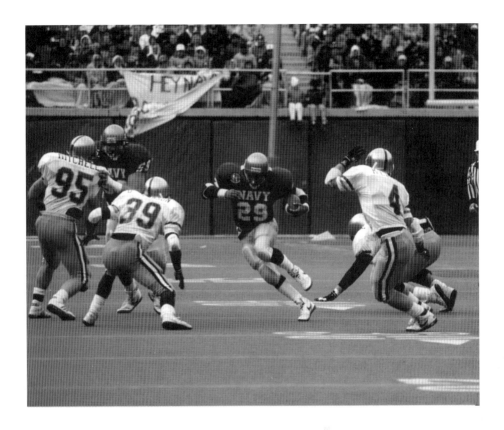

advanced study and research opportunities. In 1939, Congress bestowed the degree of B.S. upon all living graduates retroactively.

The post-World War II era to the present saw the Academy change to its present form. In 1949, the first African-American, Wesley A. Brown, graduated from the Academy.

Of the Naval Academy graduates who participated in World War II, 27 won the Congressional Medal of Honor, 18 of whom received the medal posthumously.

The Naval Academy first accepted women as midshipmen in 1976, when Congress authorized the admission of women to all of the service academies. Women comprise about 13 to 14 percent of entering

29

In terms of professional development, the Academy was up to date. The Navy's first submarine was stationed at the Academy from 1900-1915. Aviation came in 1911 with the establishment of an aerodome at Greenbury Point.

plebes—or freshmen—and they pursue the same academic and professional training as do their male classmates.

The development of the United States Naval Academy has reflected the history of the country. As America has changed culturally and tech-nologically so has the Naval Academy. In just a few decades, the Navy moved from a fleet of sail- and steam-powered ships to a high-tech fleet with nuclear-powered submarines and surface ships and supersonic aircraft. The Academy has changed, too, giving midshipmen the state-of-the-art academic and professional training they need to be effective naval officers in their future careers.

The first female Brigade Commander was Julianne Gallina, Class of 1992.

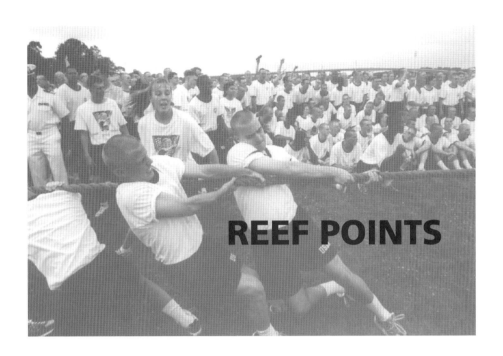

REEF POINTS

Throughout this book you will notice various facts and bits of history, lore, and color. They have been excerpted from *Reef Points*, a traditional publication of the US Naval Academy. *Reef Points* is issued to every new plebe upon arrival. If you wander the campus of the Naval Academy during plebe summer, you will notice the plebes furiously studying this book during their free time. In nautical terms, reef points are pieces of line used to reduce the area of a sail in strong winds, making for smoother sailing.

Reef Points is a small yet dense handbook containing all kinds of information. Some of it is practical, like rank insignia and rules of the sea. Some is interesting and inspiring, like the famous quotations from great Naval Officers of yesterday and today. And some is trivia and tradition. But all is expected to be read and memorized, recalled and recited, at will, upon the demand of an upperclassman, as an exercise in discipline, obedience, and brain capacity.

Here's an example:

Upperclassmen to Plebe: How long have you been in the Navy?

Plebe Response: All me bloomin' life, sir! Me mother was a mermaid, me father was King Neptune. I was born on the crest of a wave and rocked in the cradle of the deep. Seaweed and barnacles are me clothes. Every tooth in me head is a marlinspike; the hair on me head is hemp. Every bone in me body is a spar, and when I spits, I spits tar! I'se hard, I is, I am, I are!

And here's another:

Upperclassmen to Plebe: Why is There No Excuse?

Plebe Response: Sir, since I have no bombastic baccalaureate with which to create the basic augmentation of the phybitiphor, I must rely on the cooperation of the cerebrum and the medulla oblongata which compose the basis of intellectual perception. When sufficient adrenaline is not provided to cause a gagulation, then the cerebellum is placed in an inert state which brings about my position from which there is no excuse, sir.

The first vessel of note in the Navy was the *Ranger*; the first man-of-war and the first warship with the propelling machinery below the waterline was the *Princeton*; the first iron-clad, the *Monitor*; and the first submarine, the *Holland*. U.S.S. *Michigan* was our first dreadnaught; *Langley*, our first aircraft carrier, and *Nautilus* our first nuclear submarine.

Reef Points is compiled and published by the USNA's Upperclassmen. Excerpts included in this book were taken from *Reef Points 1997-1998: The Annual Handbook of the Brigade of Midshipmen, 92nd Edition.* You may want to take their advice: "A good mariner knows his instruments well; likewise, you should know this handbook from cover to cover. So remember its words and live by them."

MEET THE MIDSHIPMEN

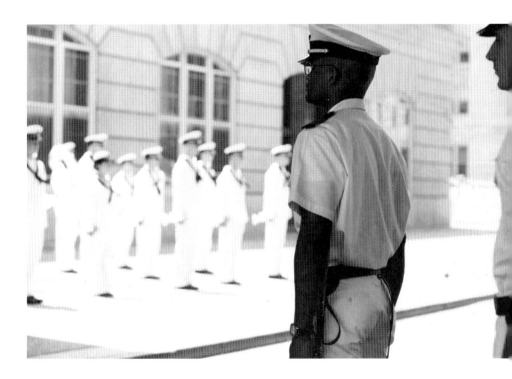

QUINTIN JONES

Quintin DeAndre Jones is a senior political science major at the Naval Academy. He hails from Memphis, Tennessee, and upon graduation will be commissioned as a second lieutenant in the United States Marine Corps. While at the Academy, he has held several positions of leadership including Plebe Summer Regimental Commander, Battalion Operations Officer, and Platoon Commander of the seventh company "Third Herd." He also participates in the Gospel Choir and is

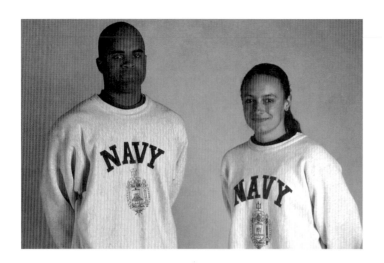

President of the Midshipman Black Studies Club. He comments, "The Naval Academy experience is what you make it, either good or bad. You can do as little or as much as you wish. The Academy also teaches humility." Other words to live by: "Push as hard as you can for as long as you can, because you would rather burn out than fade away."

JULIA MASON

Midshipman Julia Mason, a native of Linwood, NJ, is currently ranked as a Midshipman Second-Class (2/c) at the United States Naval Academy, where she has participated in the Scuba Club, Mids-for-Kids (a program in which midshipmen go out to local schools and help teachers in the classroom), and has served as a platoon sergeant and Honor Representative for her company. Midshipman Mason is also a four-time All-American swimmer and national high school champion and record-holder in the breaststroke. At the Academy, she holds pool, Academy, and Patriot League records in the 100 and 200 breast-strokes, was Patriot League swimmer of the year in 1996 and 1997, won the 100yd breaststroke at Easterns both years, and was the first female from Navy to qualify for and compete at the NCAA Division I national championships. She also enjoys reading, rowing, and hiking.

MEET THE INSTRUCTORS

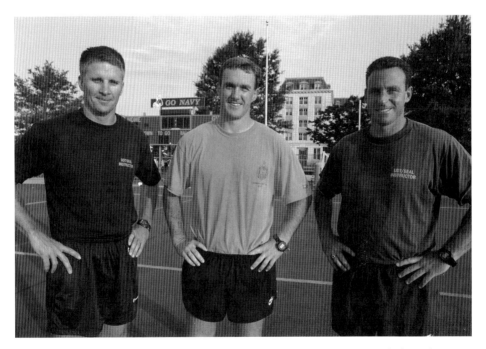

From left to right: BMC(SEAL) Walter K. Herrick, Lt. Stewart G. Smith (SEAL), and OSCS David Albonetti (SEAL).

BMC(SEAL) WALTER K. HERRICK
(BOATSWAINMATE CHIEF PETTY OFFICER)

Walter "Kirk" Herrick is a native of Manlius, New York. He has served over eighteen years in the Navy. At the age of thirty, he decided to become a SEAL. He received orders to Basic Underwater Demolition/SEAL (BUD/S) training, graduating as a member of Class 167. While in the Teams he became familiar with different types of physical fitness training programs from a wide variety of sources: BUD/S instructors, therapists, doctors, Olympic swimmers, and his teammates. After six years with the Teams, Kirk was transferred to the United States Naval Academy (USNA) as a Senior Enlisted Advisor. At USNA he has conducted swimming / water conditioning, long distance running, speed work, basic calisthenics, and strength and conditioning instruction for the four-thousand-member Brigade of Midshipmen. He is presently the Head Coach of the Women's Fastpitch Softball Team. He also coaches the Combat Pistol Team and works with several of the Varsity sports teams in their physical training. Kirk is a certified personal trainer and instructor with the Sergeant's Program in the Washington, D.C. and Annapolis, Maryland, area.

OSCS DAVID ALBONETTI (SEAL)

Operations Specialist Senior Chief Petty Officer David Albonetti led the Naval Academy physical education program for three years. Prior to his tour in Annapolis, David was stationed at SEAL Team Three. He has spent 16 years in the SEAL Teams and is a veteran of Desert Shield/ Desert Storm.

David was also selected as Senior Petty Officer of the Year for the entire Pacific Fleet. He was meritoriously promoted to Chief Petty Officer as a result of this selection.

LT. STEWART G. "STEW" SMITH (SEAL)

Lt. Stewart G. "Stew" Smith graduated from the United States Naval Academy in 1991. After graduation, he received orders to Basic Underwater Demolition/ SEAL (BUD/S) training (Class 182). While on the SEAL teams, he learned to achieve maximum levels of physical fitness thanks to the knowledge of several Chief Petty Officer SEALs, Navy doctors, and nutritionists.

After four years on the SEAL Teams, Stew was stationed at the Naval Academy and put in charge of the physical training and selection of future BUD/S students. The workouts he developed to prepare students for SEAL training are still in use today by SEAL recruiters (The BUD/S Warning Order). Stew Smith is also a certified personal trainer and instructor with the Sergeant's Program in the Washington, DC, and Annapolis, MD, area.

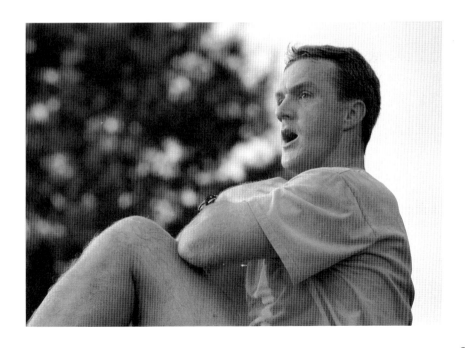

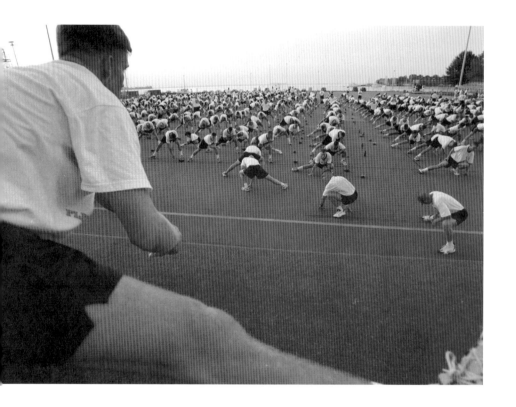

■ STRETCHES

Incorporating a proper warmup and stretching routine is essential to preventing injury and getting the maximum benefit from your work-out. You might want to start with jumping jacks, a fast walk or easy jog, and then move into the stretches. Stretching should be gentle and constant. Bouncing on your stretches only invites injury.

The stretches in this section should always be done before you start your workout. They work the major muscle groups in the upper body, abdominal region, and the lower body. When you stretch, hold each stretch on each side for 15 seconds. Do not over-stretch.

Stretching before your workout will help your body warm up. When you've completed your PT series, repeat the stretch sequence for 30 seconds per stretch on each side. This time you'll be stretching for flexibility.

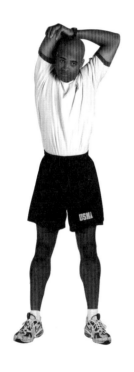 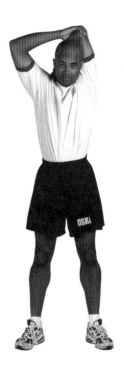

TRICEPS STRETCH

Putting your palm in the upper portion of your back between the shoulder blades, take your other hand and stretch your elbow and triceps for about 15 seconds. Switch arms. Do the stretch twice on each arm.

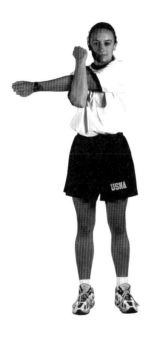 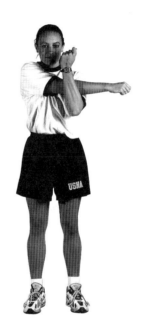

SHOULDER STRETCH

Take your right arm across your chest, putting your left arm up by your elbow. Stretch your shoulder, pulling your arm in toward your body. Hold for 15 seconds. Alternate. Do each arm twice.

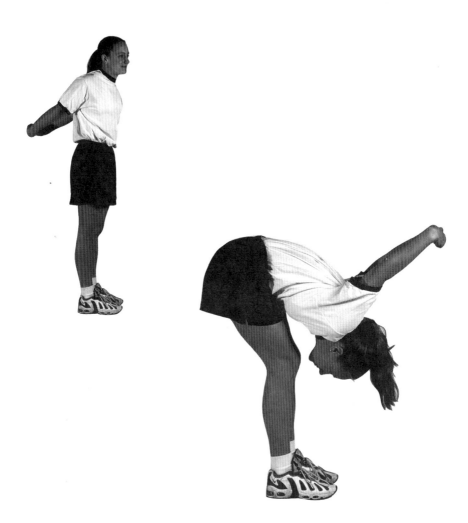

SWIMMER STRETCH

Place your feet a little more than shoulder width apart. Interlock your fingers behind your back. Bend over, bringing your hands up as far as you can. You will feel your back stretching. Keep your legs straight. This will stretch out your shoulders and hamstrings too.

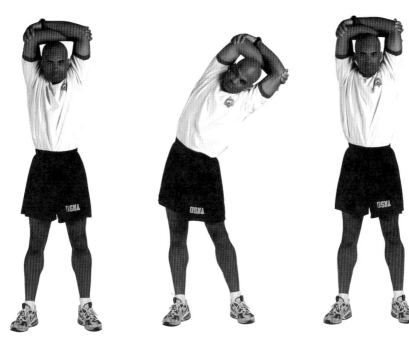

TRUNK SIDE STRETCH

Place your arms on top of your head and grab your elbows, then gently bend to the left, stretching out your torso. Return to starting position. Then stretch to your right side. Return to starting position. TAKE THE FIRST 4 COUNTS SLOWLY. Hold each count for about 5 or 10 seconds. Then make it into a quicker 4-count exercise.

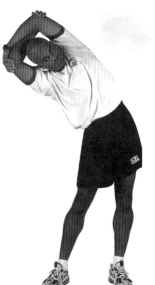

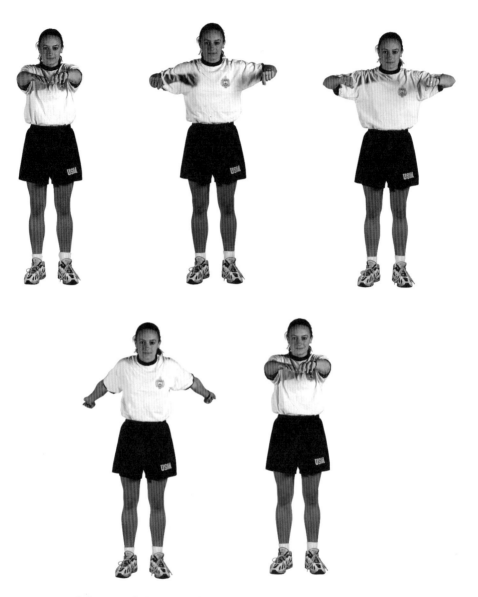

PRESS-PRESS-FLING

This stretch will definitely loosen up your chest. Hold your arms shoulder height, parallel to the floor. Arms bent at a 90 degree angle. Pull back 2 times nice and easy. On third count...end with a clap. There is constant motion. No stopping.

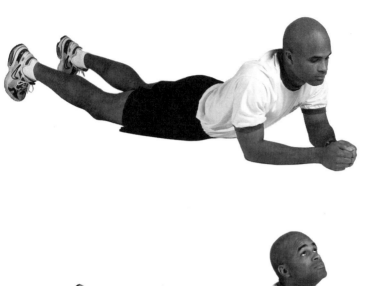

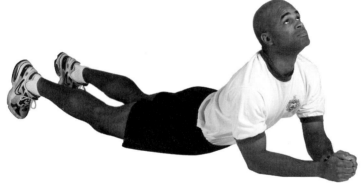

STOMACH STRETCH (ABDOMEN)

Lay flat on your stomach with your elbows underneath your chest. Keep your elbows on the deck and your feet flat on the ground. This is an easy stretch for abs and lower back. Raise up gently as shown for about 10 seconds, being careful not to overstretch your lower back. Relax down to the starting position. Repeat this stretch 4 or 5 times. BE CAREFUL NOT TO OVERSTRETCH!

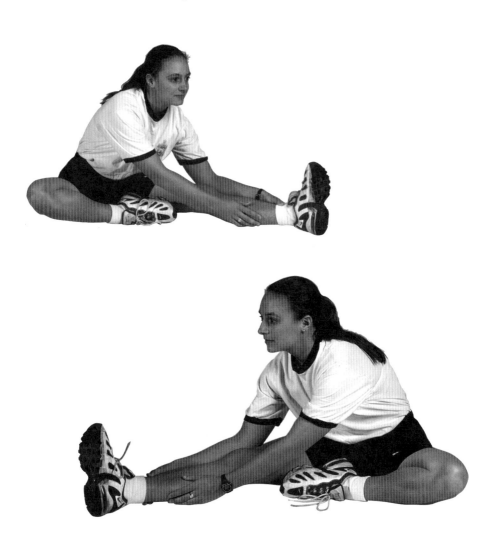

HURDLER STRETCH

Sitting on the deck, extend your left leg and bring your right foot to the inner part of your left thigh as shown in the photo. Keeping your back straight and head up, gently grab your ankle. Keep your arms relaxed and do not bounce. You will feel a constant pull on your hamstring. Hold this position for about 10 seconds; then relax. Do 3 to 4 repetitions on each side.

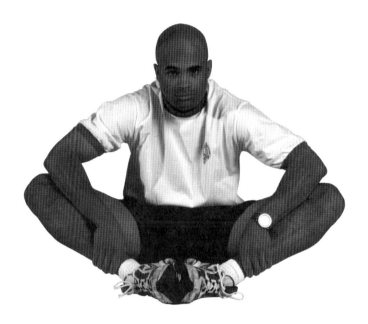

BUTTERFLIES

Bring your feet and heels in, grabbing ankles. Put constant, gentle pressure on the inside of your knees and press down. Hold for a count of ten. Release and relax. Repeat 4 or 5 times. Again, avoid the temptation to bounce. You might want to gently rock side to side to work the stretch around.

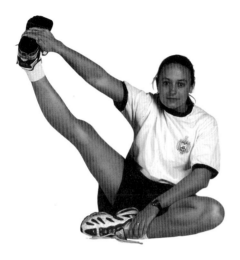

HAMSTRING STRETCH

Bring your left leg in and grab your right foot on the instep, bringing it up. Straighten your leg out as much as you can. If you can't straighten your leg, that's OK. Maximum flexibility takes time and many repetitions to achieve. Each stretch is a 10-second count, then a release. Do 4 repetitions on each side.

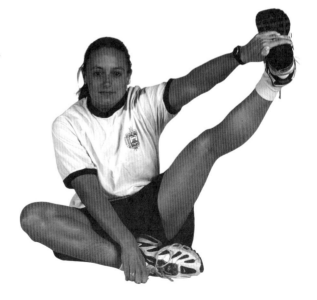

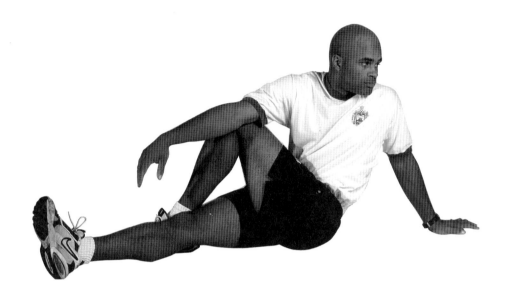

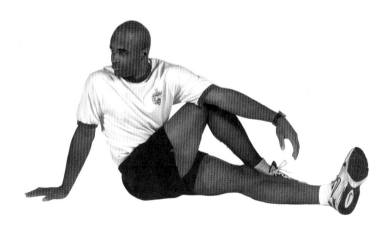

LOWER BACK STRETCH

Take your right leg and place it over your left knee. Then take your right elbow and place it inside your right knee. Slowly exhale and twist to the left. Turn your head to the left as well. Repeat on the right side, switching legs.

49

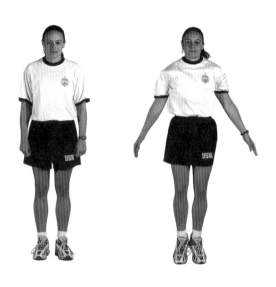

JUMPING JACKS 4 COUNT

The jumping jack is a classic cardio warmup and conditioning exercise. This exercise is a 4-count calisthenics activity—two jumping jacks are counted as one. One, two, three, ONE. One, two, three, TWO. A standard warmup would include 25 counted jumping jack repetitions prior to stretching.

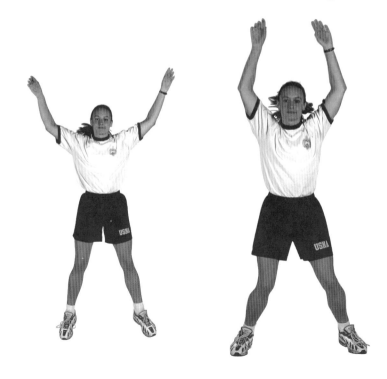

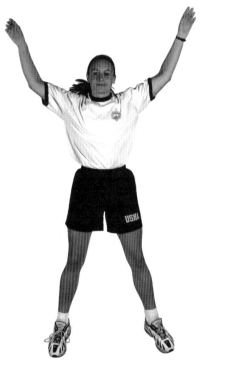

No United States warship has ever mutinied or been in the hands of mutineers.

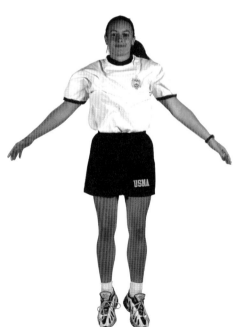

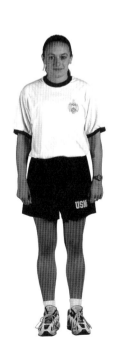

51

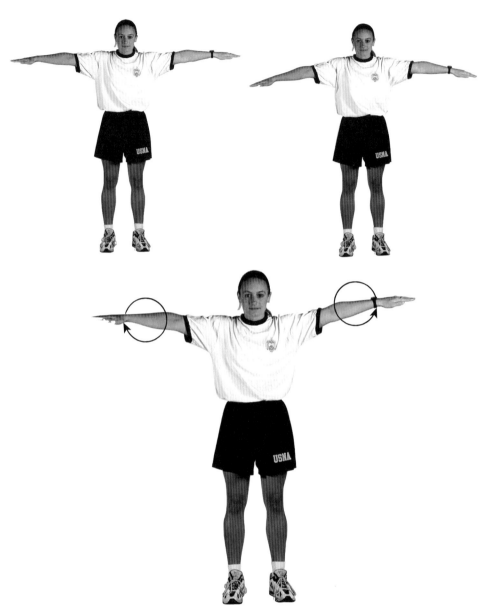

ARM CIRCLES

This stretch is excellent for working your shoulders. Keep your palms down, starting by making small circles to the front for 30 seconds. Then do small circles to the side for 30 secs. When you start to feel

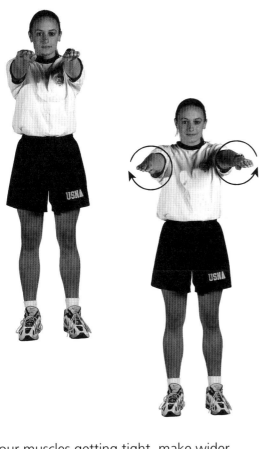

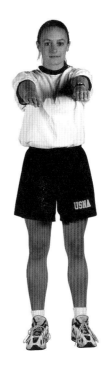

your muscles getting tight, make wider circles. To vary this warmup, you can change the position of your hands, alternating between palms up and down, as well as alternating the direction of your arms from the front to the side, to above your head, as shown on the next page.

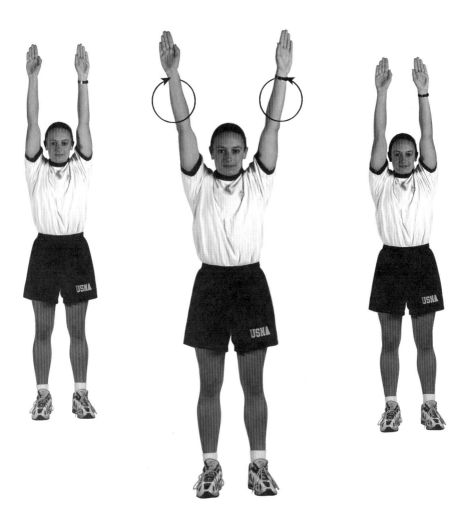

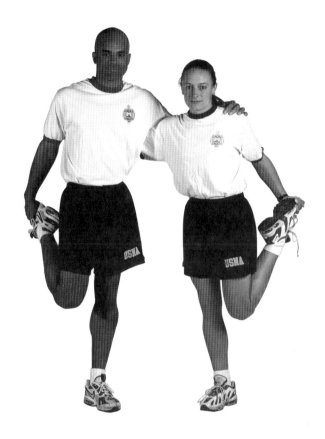

THIGH STRETCH STANDING

Standing on one leg, grab your foot behind you and gently lift it to your buttocks. Hold the stretch for the required length and release. Switch legs. You may need hold onto a wall to keep your balance, or you can lean against your workout partner as shown in the photo above.

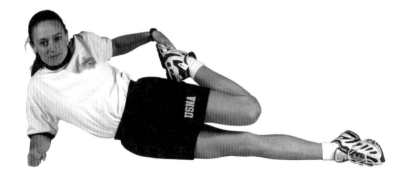

THIGH STRETCH PRONE

This stretch is an alternative to the Thigh Stretch Standing, and is especially useful when there is no object or person to lean against. Lying on your side, grab your foot as shown and pull it toward your buttocks. Hold and release the stretch gently. Switch sides and repeat.

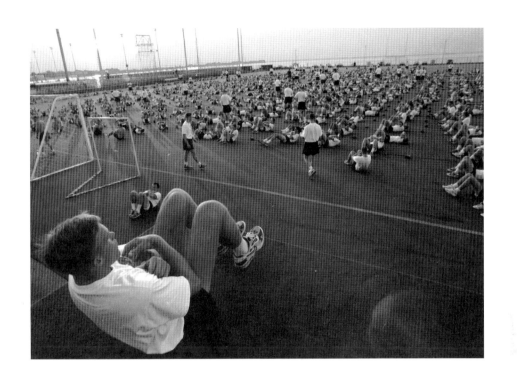

UPPER BODY
EXERCISES

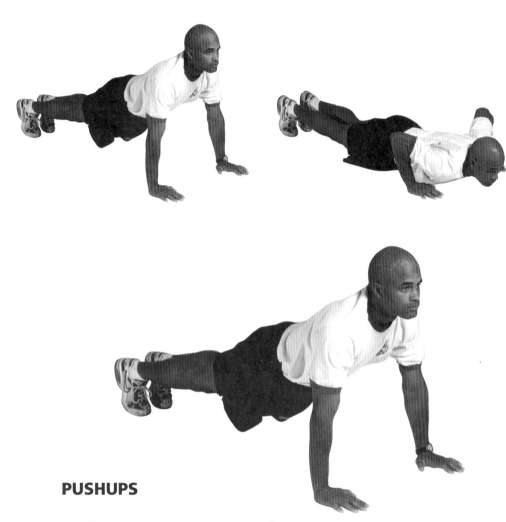

PUSHUPS

A military P.T. classic. Learn to perform this exercise properly for maximum benefit. You'll be working your upper chest in this exercise. Keep your back straight and your feet together, hands a bit more than shoulder width apart. Make sure you practice good posture, keeping your back nice and straight. Push down and touch your chest to the deck, remembering always to keep your back straight. This is a 2-count exercise. Down-up. One. Down-up. Two.

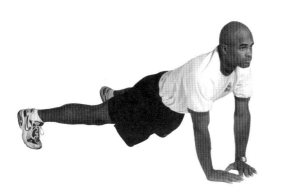

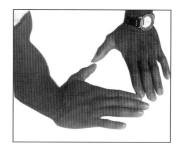

Detail

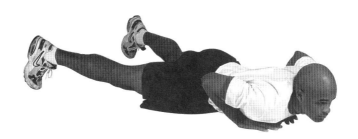

TRICEPS PUSHUPS

Legs are spread wider than shoulder length. Make a diamond with your hands as shown. Keep your back straight. The object when doing these pushups is to do the exercises with proper form, slowly and methodically, so you work the muscles efficiently. Speed does not matter as much as technique. Concentrate on keeping your back straight.

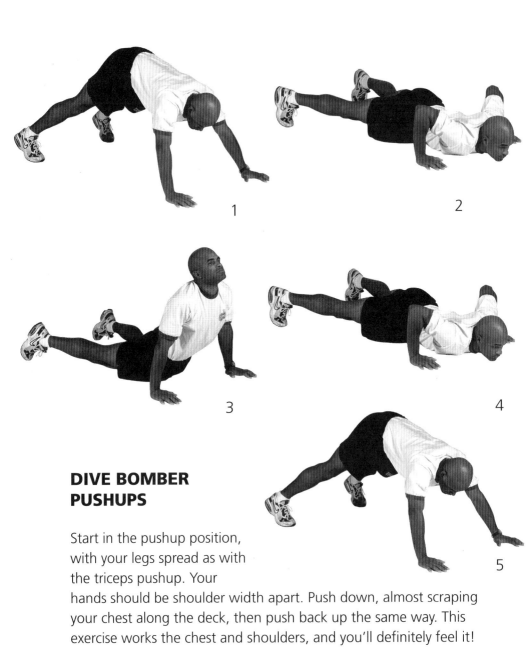

1

2

3

4

DIVE BOMBER PUSHUPS

Start in the pushup position, with your legs spread as with the triceps pushup. Your

5

hands should be shoulder width apart. Push down, almost scraping your chest along the deck, then push back up the same way. This exercise works the chest and shoulders, and you'll definitely feel it!

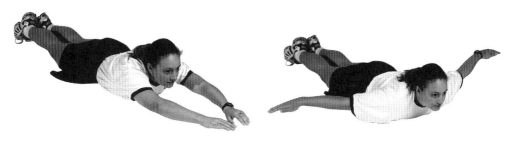

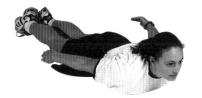

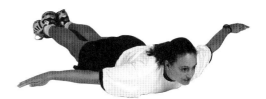

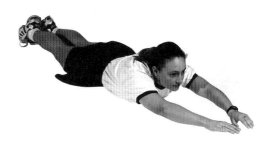

ARM HAULERS

Lie down on the deck with your
feet about shoulder width apart
but not touching the deck. Arms
should start at your sides. In one
motion, swing your arms up from
your sides to straight over your head as shown and back down to
your sides again. This is great for your shoulders and upper back
muscles.

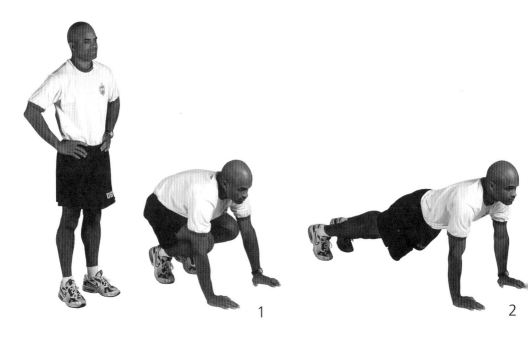

1

2

EIGHT COUNT BODY BUILDERS

The 8-Count Body Builder is a unique exercise combining a variety of moves and muscles. The result is a powerful exercise that works the upper body, lower body, and cardiorespiratory system.

Here's how you do it. Begin in a standing position. Move to a squat position with your arms slightly more than shoulder width apart and count "1." Thrust your legs straight back, count "2." Keeping your back straight, lower yourself in a picture perfect pushup "3" and up "4." Kick your legs apart like a scissor "5," then kick them back together "6." Pull your legs back in a reverse thrust motion "7." And stand "8." You have just performed one 8-Count Body Builder.

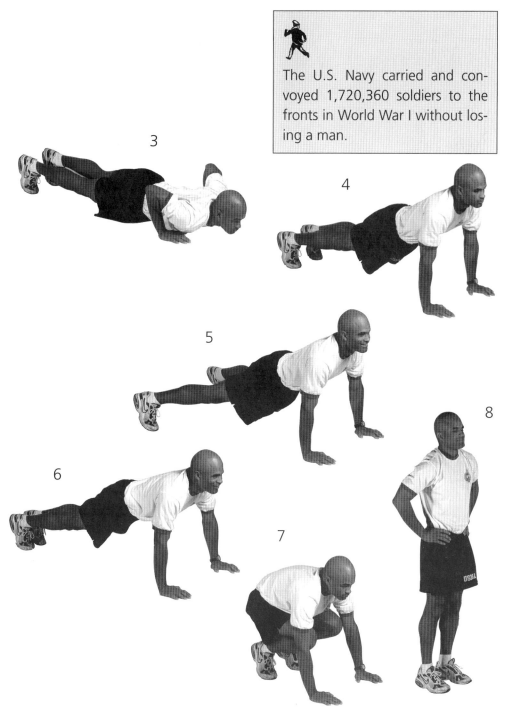

The U.S. Navy carried and convoyed 1,720,360 soldiers to the fronts in World War I without losing a man.

3

4

5

8

6

7

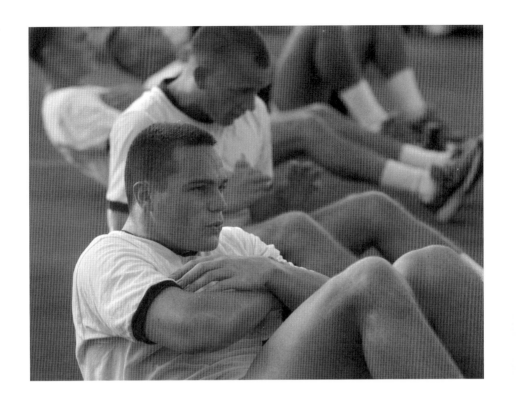

ABDOMINAL EXERCISES

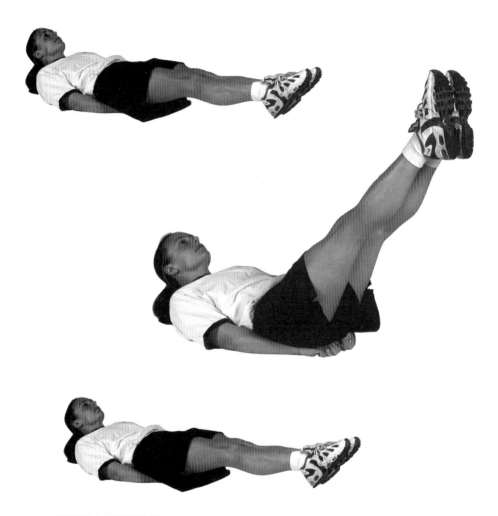

LEG LEVERS

Lie flat on the ground with your hands underneath your buttocks. Legs should be straight and toes pointed. Lift your legs up from about 6 inches to 36 inches. Count 1. Bring them back down and count 2. This exercise works the hip flexors and lower abs. If your lower back hurts doing leg levers, you can hold on to a partner's legs if they stand behind you. This will help keep your back flat as well.

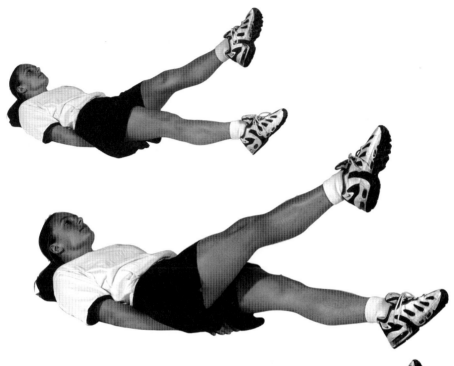

FLUTTER KICKS

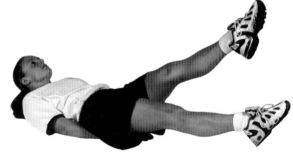

Lie flat on the ground with your hands underneath your buttocks. Legs should be straight and toes pointed. This is a 4-count exercise. Move one leg at a time from 6 inches to 36 inches. This works your abdominals somewhat but mostly works hip flexors. Flutter kicks are used a lot by SEAL teams to condition them for intense amounts of swimming.

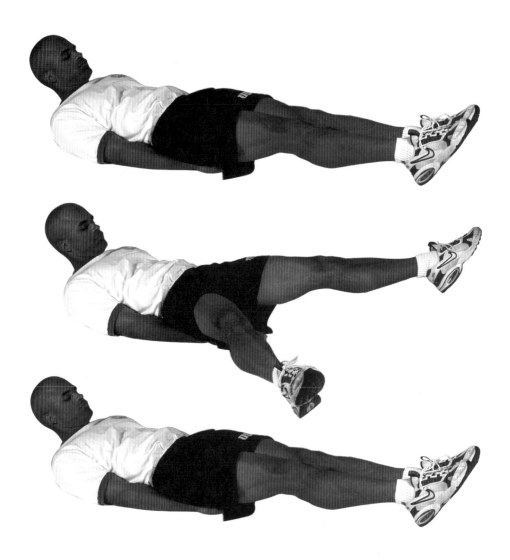

SCISSORS

Place your hands underneath your buttocks and position your feet straight out. Toes should be pointed. With your legs about 6 inches off the deck, open then close your legs in a scissor-like motion. This is a 2-count exercise.

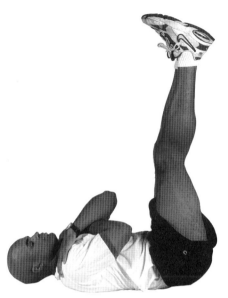
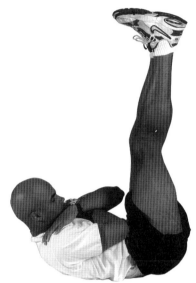

AB CRUNCHES: MODIFICATION 1

Put your legs straight up in the air with your hands across your chest. Bring your shoulder blades off the deck and contract your stomach. It doesn't matter how high you lift your shoulders or how fast you do each crunch; it's most important to come up and hold for a 2-count. Always exhale on the way up. Take a breath on the way down. It's a little harder when your legs are up in the

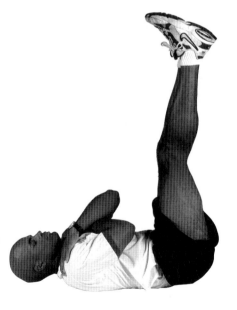

air; not only are you doing the crunch but you're using your stomach muscles to keep your legs in the air as well. You should hold each crunch for a count of 2 but try to hold it for a count of 6 or even 15.

69

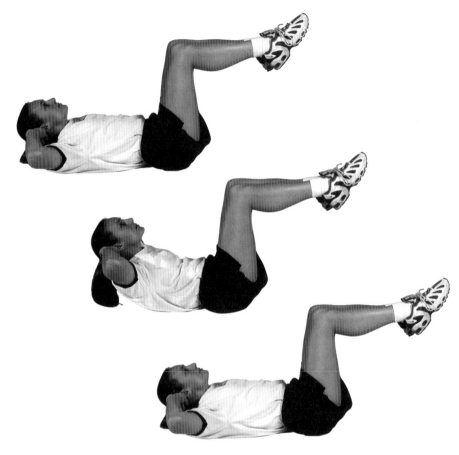

AB CRUNCHES: MODIFICATION 2

Put your feet up at a 90 degree angle. Put your hands behind your head but don't interlock your fingers; just let them touch each other. You don't want to put a strain on your neck. Curl up and contract your stomach, exhaling on the way up and taking a breath on the way down. When you put your hands on your head think of your head as a very ripe melon. You don't want to crush it. You don't want to hyperextend your neck. Try for a deliberately slow, controlled action.

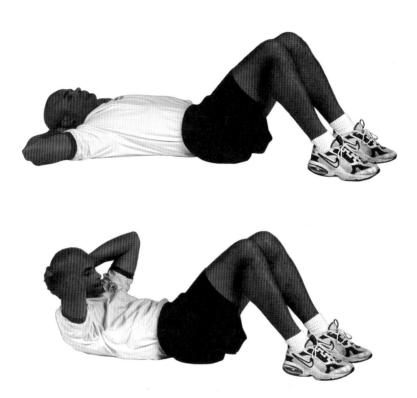

AB CRUNCHES: MODIFICATION 3 (ADVANCED)

Starting position is flat on your back. Arms should be behind your head, feet and knees together. Curl up, getting your shoulders off the deck. It doesn't matter how far up you go; it's how hard you contract your stomach that counts. This exercise really tones your abs. Hold each crunch for 2 counts, and then return to the starting position.

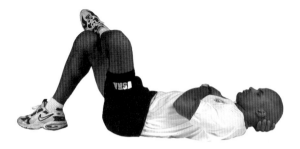

The youngest midshipman was Samuel Baron, appointed from Virginia at the age of two.

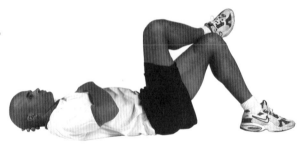

AB CRUNCHES: MODIFICATION 4

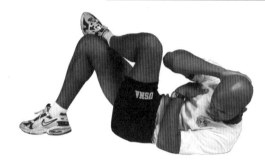

This definitely works your obliques and abs. Your left hand should be out to your side or across your chest. Place your right-hand palm against your ear. Raise up and bring your right elbow to-wards your left knee. Once again, you don't have to touch. You want to get a good contraction of your

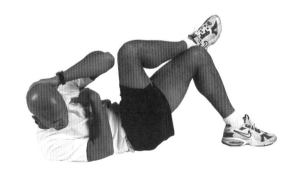

abs. Do this crunch on both sides and remember: don't pull up on your neck!

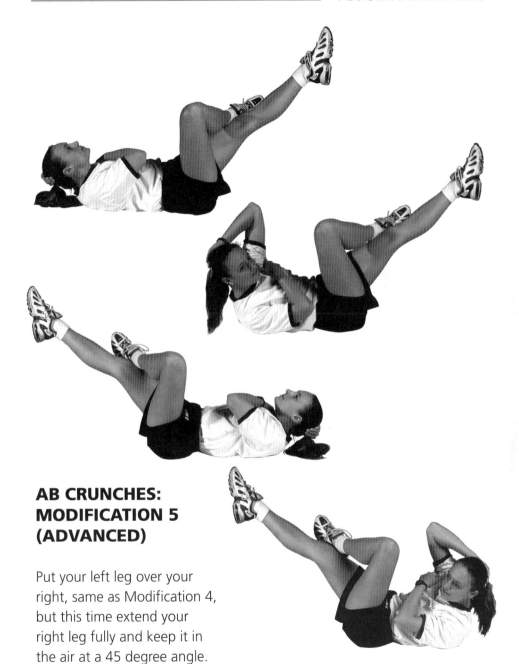

AB CRUNCHES: MODIFICATION 5 (ADVANCED)

Put your left leg over your right, same as Modification 4, but this time extend your right leg fully and keep it in the air at a 45 degree angle. This puts constant pressure on your abs. If you put your left hand in your armpit, the only thing supporting you is your abs and your back. This is a very advanced crunch.

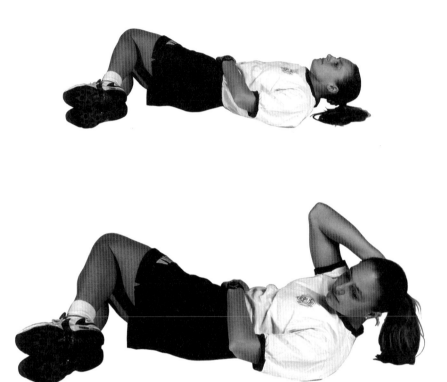

OBLIQUE CRUNCH 1

This crunch works the side muscles of your abdominal section, or the oblique muscles. Laying on your side as shown, one hand behind your neck and the other across your waist, lift your shoulder off the deck while contracting your oblique muscles. Avoid twisting and try to keep your motion on a single plane. Tighten up, contract your abs, then release and relax. Repeat.

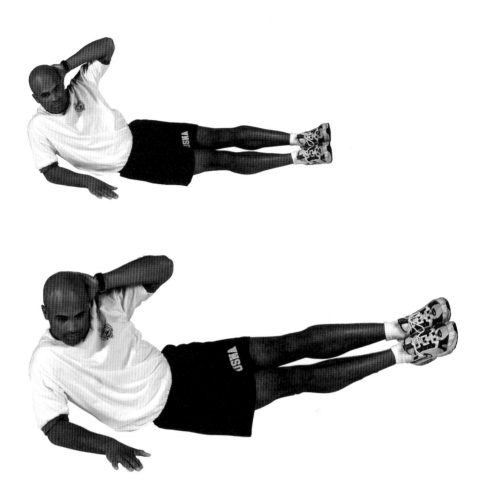

OBLIQUE CRUNCH 2: LOW OBLIQUE RAISE

Lay down on your left side for this 2-count exercise. Legs should be straight, feet together. Your left arm should also be straight. Place your right hand on your ear. Come up and contract obliques. Go from 2-10 inches off the deck. You only need a slight movement for the crunch. Do this exercise on the left side and then alternate, concentrating on the right side.

75

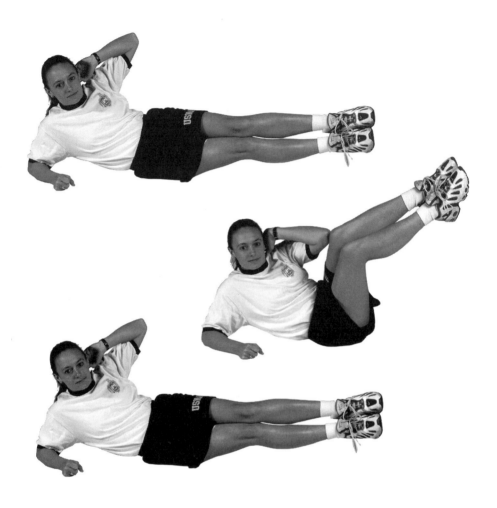

OBLIQUE CRUNCH 3: HIGH OBLIQUE RAISE

Place one hand under your body, and the other hand behind your head. Your feet should be about 6 inches off the deck. Legs straight, toes pointed. Position your head at a 45 degree angle. Bring your feet from 6 inches to 36 inches and touch your elbow to your knees.

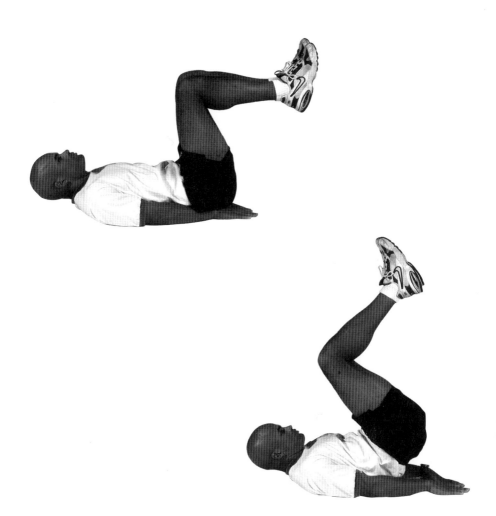

REVERSE CRUNCH

Lay on your back with your legs up in the air and bent at the knees. Bring your knees in toward your chest, while lifting your lower back and buttocks off the deck. Return to the starting position and repeat. As with all crunches, it's technique that counts most, so do them right!

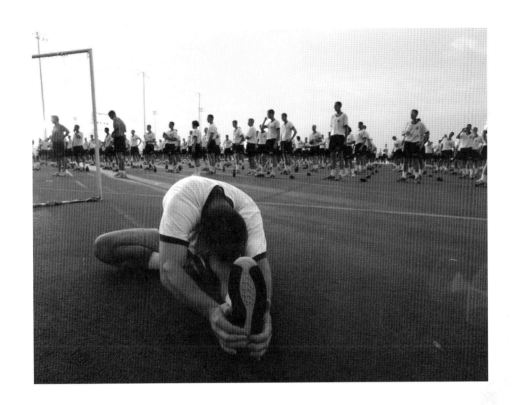

LOWER BODY
EXERCISES

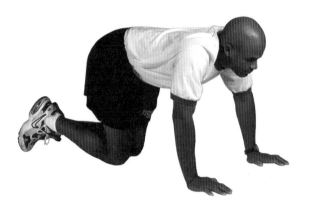

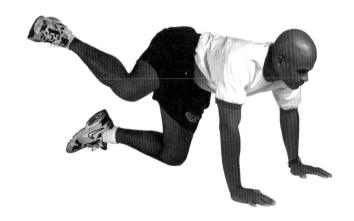

SIDE LEG LIFT

This exercise is often referred to as the "Dirty Dog." Crouching on your hands and knees (as shown in the photo), lift your left leg to your side and bring it back down again. Count that as one repetition. Perform the specified number of repetitions and switch sides. The Side Leg Lift is excellent for strengthening and toning thighs, hips, and buttocks.

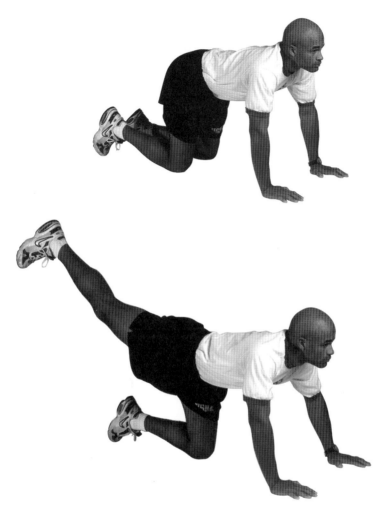

REAR LEG LIFT

The starting position is identical to the Side Leg Lift; however, this exercise is conducted by extending your leg directly to the rear and upward, in a kick-like motion. This exercise is also referred to as the "Donkey Kick." Perform the specified number of repetitions on each side according to your workout schedule.

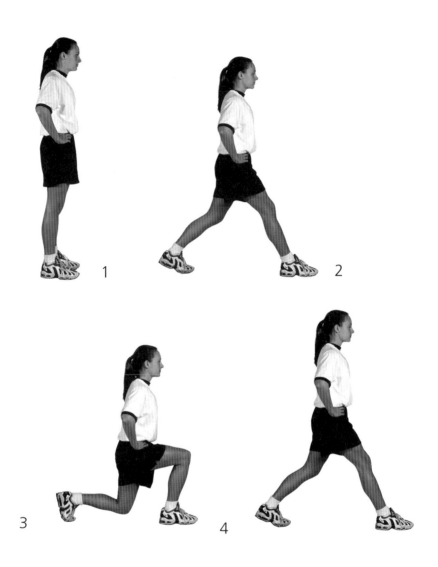

LUNGES

Step forward with your right leg as shown. Bend your front knee until a 90 degree angle is formed with your right leg, being careful not to lean too far forward! Keep your knee directly above your ankle during the downward movement to avoid overstressing the knee joint.

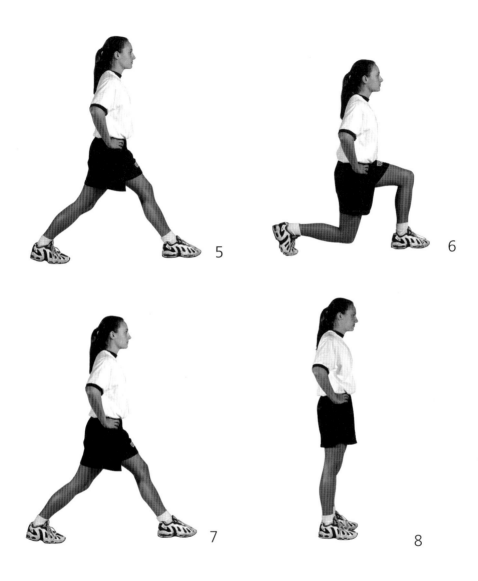

Repeat the lunge with the other leg forward after you have performed the specified number of repetitions. Your thighs, hamstrings, and buttocks all benefit from this exercise.

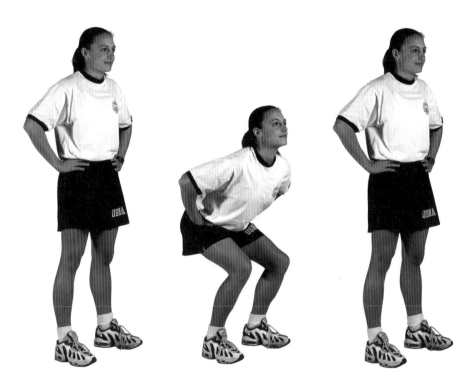

SQUATS

Stand with your legs about shoulder width apart. With your head up and back straight, bend at your knees until a 90 degree angle is formed with your legs. Slowly lift yourself to standing position and repeat. Squats are a great lower body exercise and work thighs, hamstrings, and buttocks.

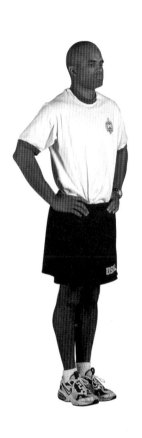 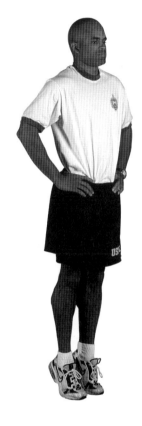

The width of the Panama Canal formerly determined the beam of a United States naval vessel; the Brooklyn Bridge, its height.

TWO-LEG CALF RAISE

Calf Raises are excellent for developing strong calf muscles and aid in developing balance strength by exercising the stabilizer muscles in your lower leg. To perform the Two-Leg Calf Raise, stand flat footed with feet together as shown. Lift yourself up and then lower yourself down, on your toes only.

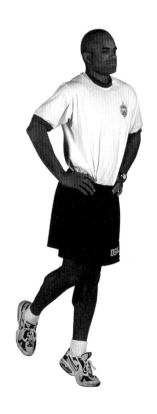

SINGLE LEG CALF RAISE VARIATION

Lift one foot off the floor. Lift yourself up your toes—keep your balance! This variation is more difficult because you are placing more weight on the single calf muscle. Strength and balance are both developed in this advanced exercise. To maintain your balance, you can lean on your workout buddy, or against a wall. Try to build up your balance strength so you can perform this exercise unassisted.

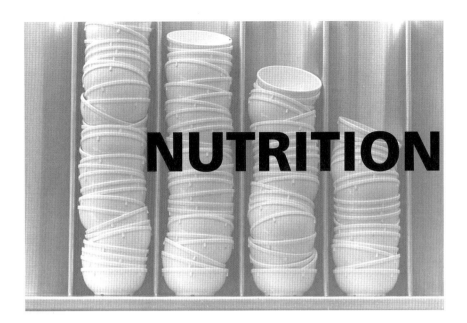

NUTRITION

Y ou can't achieve peak physical fitness without paying attention to what you eat. Strong dietary habits are critical both before entering the Academy and during Academy training as well. Optimum performance is achieved by proper nutrient intake and is essential to receiving maximum performance output during exercise. Nutrition also promotes vital muscle and tissue growth and repair. The ideal diet provides all the nutrients that the body needs and supplies energy for exercise.

The Navy has developed a nutrition and weight control program to enable participants to vastly improve their health and fitness. The program deals with excess body fat and highlights the foods that will be most effective in helping you achieve your personal fitness goals. Used in conjunction with this or any physical conditioning regimen, this nutrition program will help you maintain and improve your health.

The following information on nutrition is essential for adopting healthy eating and exercise habits. Although the program is designed primarily as a weight management education tool, the Navy recommends it to all Midshipmen for the maintenance of long-term optimum health. The nutrition and diet program is successful only when used in conjunction with a physical conditioning program and is not to be used as a one-time, "quick fix" diet.

For example, a weight-loss program that reduces fat and incorporates complex carbohydrates but does not include exercise will ultimately fail. Similarly, increased exercise without a carefully monitored calorie intake will bring disappointing results. You need to consume a great amount of complex carbohydrates to provide the energy you need to sustain a strenuous physical program at the Academy.

A healthy body fat percentage for men is 14 to 16 percent; for women, 24 to 26 percent.

Before starting a nutrition or a weight-control program, it is essential to understand the way our bodies process the foods we eat.

WHAT IS NUTRITION?

Nutrition is the science of nourishment, the study of nutrients and the process by which organisms use them. In other words, nutrition is the way our bodies get energy from the food we eat. So the old saying, "You are what you eat" may not be far from the truth, considering the performance of the body is directly related to how we fuel ourselves. The study of nutrition has proven that poor nutritional habits have a profound effect on physical and mental capabilities and affect all functions of the body. Without the most fundamental of nutrients, including water, the body quickly begins to deteriorate.

Good nutrition is fundamental to every living organism on the earth in order to grow and function properly. There are six nutrients derived from food: carbohydrates, protein, and fat, which provide the body with calories; and vitamins, minerals, and water, which provide no calories. It is important to note

After exhaustive exercise, it takes at least 20 hours to completely restore muscle energy.

that while carbohydrates and proteins supply the body with four calories each per gram, fat contributes nine calories per gram—more than double. Therefore, it is important to monitor fat intake when maintaining or losing weight. Similarly, a diet and exercise program must incorporate carbohydrates that provide the body with the energy needed to sustain an exercise regimen.

Carbohydrates are sugars and starches in food and are derived from the plant kingdom. Typically, carbohydrates are called either simple or complex and provide the body with most of its fuel. Examples of complex carbohydrates include bread, rice, pasta, potatoes, cereals, and whole grains. Simple carbohydrates include fruits and vegetables. Refined simple sugars are found in candy, cakes, cookies, sodas, etc. and provide a quick source of energy. Some carbohydrates, such as fruits and vegetables, are also rich in dietary fiber, another chief element of a healthy diet.

A high carbohydrate diet is essential to maintaining energy during heavy training.

Dietary fiber is found only in plant food and is the "indigestible" part of the plant. So although fiber is edible, it is not digested or absorbed by humans. Similarly, fiber itself is calorie-free although typically foods rich in fiber usually contain calories. Fiber is made up of two types: soluble and insoluble. Soluble fiber lowers cholesterol levels. Its sources include fruits and vegetables, especially apples, oranges, carrots, oat bran, barley, and beans. Insoluble fiber increases the bulk of food thereby speeding the passage of food through the digestive tract. Insoluble fiber is found in fruits with edible skins, whole grains and breads, and whole grain cereals. Although 25 to 30 grams of fiber per day is recommended, statistics show that most Americans fail to consume this recommended daily allowance and take in only 10 to 15 grams per day.

Protein is essential to the human body. Protein functions to repair and build tissues, provide a structural role in all body tissues and contributes to the formation of enzymes, hormones, and antibodies. Protein consists of amino acids that are sometimes called the "building blocks" of protein. Protein in the diet is broken down into amino acids during digestion. Complete proteins are foods containing large amounts of essential amino acids. Complete proteins are found in animal proteins including beef, chicken, pork, fish, eggs, milk, and cheese. There are also incomplete proteins, which, as their name implies, are deficient in one or more of the eight essential amino acids. Incomplete proteins are derived from non-animal sources such as legumes including soybeans, peanuts, peas, beans and lentils, grains, and vegetables.

Fat. Perhaps the most talked about issue recently has been the presence of fat in our diets. Fat comes from the oils found in food and is stored in the body as triglycerides, which are more commonly known as body fat. Fat is found in vegetable oils, butter, shortening, lard, margarine, and animal foods such as beef, chicken, and diary products. The popular misconception is that all fat is bad. Adults require a minimum of 15 to 25 grams of fat daily. Fat manufactures antibodies to fight disease, serves as carriers of certain vitamins, protects vital organs, and insulates the body against environmental temperature changes. In addition, fat lines and insulates neurons or nerves, which allow all neural information to move through the brain and the body. We would not be able to move or think without the presence of fat. There are three different kinds of fat: polyunsaturated, monosaturated, and saturated.

FINDING THE RIGHT BALANCE

How does all of this translate to our personal fitness and weight loss? Remember that while carbohydrates and proteins produce only 4 calories per gram, fat provides the body with 9 calories per gram. There are 3,500 calories on one pound of fat tissue. When someone consumes 3,500 calories more than they burn, they gain one pound of fat. Similarly, when they use 3,500 calories more than they consume, they lose one pound of fat. A healthy body fat percentage for men is 14 to 16 percent; for women, 24 to 26 percent.

Although all three—carbohydrates, protein, and fat—are sources of energy nutrients, carbohydrates are the preferred source of energy for physical activity. After exhaustive exercise, it takes at least 20 hours to completely restore muscle energy, assuming that 600 grams of carbohydrates are consumed per day. A high carbohydrate diet is essential to maintaining energy during successive days of heavy training when energy stores before each training session become progressively lower.

The popular misconception is that all fat is bad.

The best sources of complex carbohydrates are bread, crackers, cereal, beans, pasta, potatoes, rice, fruits, and vegetables. *You should consume at least four servings of these food groups per day when training.*

Stay hydrated. In addition, frequent water intake is crucial. It is important to stay hydrated and consume water prior to feeling thirsty. Drink at least four quarts of water daily, staying away from alcohol, caffeine, and tobacco, which increase your body's need for water.

Good nutritional habits should not be limited to a specified training period but must become a lifetime commitment. Although we have been conditioned to think that eating three square meals per day is healthy, ideally calories should be spread evenly throughout the day with smaller meals that may occur three, four, five, or six times a day. The amount of meals and the numbers of hours in between eating should be based on each particular lifestyle.

Although conditioned to eat three meals a day, ideally we should get calories from smaller meals spread evenly throughout the day.

Skipping meals, especially breakfast, is strongly inadvisable. According to research, approximately 90 percent of people with a weight problem skip at least one or two meals daily with breakfast being the most frequently missed. Skipping meals causes the metab-

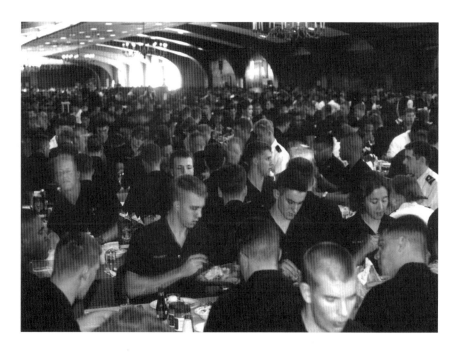

olism to lower itself to conserve energy. It also promotes overeating in the evening after a meal has been skipped during the day. However, research shows that metabolism increases by 50 percent after eating breakfast.

Metabolism increases by 50 percent after eating breakfast.

It is strongly recommended that you keep a log of everything you have consumed, including fluids, during the day. Record each meal or snack along with the time of day. In this way, your progress will be accurately marked and serve as a vital tool in advancing your physical state of well-being.

6-WEEK WORKOUT AND FITNESS PLAN

D esigned to assist in meeting the NAVY PRT requirements which are:

	Men	Women
Pushups	No less than 40	No less than 18
Curl-ups*	No less than 65	No less than 65
Timed 1.5-mile Run	No greater than 10 min. 30 sec.	No greater than 12 min. 38 sec.

* A curl-up is performed as follows: Lie flat on the back; flex knees, thighs 45 degrees to deck, legs shoulder width apart, heels not more than 10 inches from the buttocks, arms folded across chest, hands touching shoulders. Feet flat on the deck are held by a partner only on insteps. From starting position, curl-up until the head is directly above knees. When shoulder blades touch the deck, one repetition has been completed. Do as many repetitions as possible in two minutes.

THE USNA PHYSICAL EDUCATION PROGRAM (P.E.P.) 6-WEEK WORKOUT AND FITNESS PLAN

The Physical Education Program (P.E.P.) is an integral part of the Plebe Summer Indoctrination process which brings the plebes to an acceptable level of fitness, while instructing them in personal conditioning and building teamwork and spirit through challenging physical activity.

The P.E.P. regimen is a progressive workout. Those participating in P.E.P. are reminded that P.E.P. is designed to challenge the average 18-21 year old student physically and teach military P.T. and running programs.

WEEK # 1

MONDAY	TUESDAY	WEDNESDAY
UPPER BODY	LOWER BODY PT	TAKE A DAY OFF AND REST!

Warmup: 1/4 mile jog

Stretch: 10 min.

Pushups	Reps
Regular	20
Triceps	15
Dive Bomber	10
8-Count	10
Arm Haulers	40

Abdominals

Curl-ups	50
Crunches	20
Flutter Kicks	25
Leg Levers	25

Platoon Run
1.5 miles

Warmup: 1/4 mile jog

Stretch: 10 min.

Legs	
Squats	15
Lunges	15
Calf Raises	20
Sprints	50m
	75m
	100m

Abdominals

Curl-ups	2 x 50
Crunches	4 x 40
Flutter Kicks	30
Leg Levers	30

Platoon Run
1.5 miles

Words of encouragement:

"Hit hard, hit fast, hit often."
—Admiral "Bull" Halsey's battle cry

WEEK # 1

THURSDAY	FRIDAY	SATURDAY

LOWER BODY PT | UPPER BODY PT | LOWER BODY PT

Warmup: 1/4 mile jog | **Warmup:** 1/4 mile jog | **Warmup:** 1/4 mile jog

Stretch: 10 min. | **Stretch:** 10 min. | **Stretch:** 10 min.

THURSDAY — Lower Body PT

Legs
Squats	3 x 15
Lunges	3 x 15
Calf Raises	3 x 20
Sprints	50m
	75m
	100m

Abdominals
Timed Curl-ups
40 in 1 min. x 2
30 in 45 sec.
20 in 30 sec.
Crunches	4 x 40
Flutter Kicks	30
Leg Levers	30

Platoon Run
1.5 miles

FRIDAY — Upper Body PT

Pushups	**Reps**
Regular	4 x 20
Triceps	4 x 15
Dive Bomber	15
8-Count	15
Arm Hauler	40

Abdominals
| Curl-ups | 50 |
| Crunches | 20 |

Platoon Run
1.5 miles

SATURDAY — Lower Body PT

Legs
Squats	3 x 15
Lunges	3 x 15
Calf Raises	3 x 20
Sprints	50m
	75m
	100m

Abdominals
Timed Curl-ups
40 in 1 min. x 2
30 in 45 sec. x 2
20 in 30 sec.
Crunches	4 x 40
Flutter Kicks	25
Leg Levers	25

95

WEEK # 2

MONDAY	TUESDAY	WEDNESDAY
UPPER BODY PT	LOWER BODY PT	TAKE A DAY OFF AND REST!

MONDAY

UPPER BODY PT

Warmup: 1/4 mile jog

Stretch: 10 min.

Pushups	Reps
Regular	3 x 20
Triceps	3 x 15
Dive Bomber	3 x 10
8-Count	2 x 10
Arm Haulers	2 x 40

Abdominals

Curl-ups	50 x 2
Crunches	20 x 2
Flutter Kicks	25 x 2
Leg Levers	25 x 2
Timed Situps	
30 sec. x 2 (goal 20)	
45 sec. x 2 (goal 30)	

Platoon Run
2 miles

TUESDAY

LOWER BODY PT

Warmup: 1/4 mile jog

Stretch: 10 min.

Legs	Reps
Squats	3 x 15
Lunges	3 x 15
Calf Raises	3 x 20
Sprints	3 x 50m
	3 x 75m
	3 x 100m
Dirty Dogs	3 x 40

Platoon Run
2 miles

WEDNESDAY

TAKE A DAY OFF AND REST!

Words of encouragement:

"He who will not risk cannot win."
—*John Paul Jones*

WEEK # 2

THURSDAY	FRIDAY	SATURDAY
UPPER BODY PT	LOWER BODY PT	UPPER BODY PT

THURSDAY — UPPER BODY PT

Warmup: 1/4 mile jog

Stretch: 10 min.

Pushups	Reps
Regular	3 x 20
Triceps	3 x 15
Dive Bomber	3 x 10
8-Count	2 x 10
Arm Haulers	2 x 40

Abdominals	
Curl-ups	50 x 2
Crunches	20 x 2
Flutter Kicks	25 x 2
Leg Levers	25 x 2
Timed Situps	
30 sec. x 2 (goal 20)	
45 sec. x 2 (goal 30)	

Platoon Run
2 miles

FRIDAY — LOWER BODY PT

Warmup: 1/4 mile jog

Stretch: 10 min.

Legs	Reps
Squats	3 x 15
Lunges	3 x 15
Calf Raises	3 x 20
Sprints	3 x 50m
	3 x 75m
	3 x 100m
Dirty Dogs	3 x 40

Platoon Run
2 miles

SATURDAY — UPPER BODY PT

Warmup: 1/4 mile jog

Stretch: 10 min.

Pyramid Workout

```
              20
          18 /\ 18
         16 /    \ 16
        14 /      \ 14
       12 /        \ 12
      10 /          \ 10
       8 /            \ 8
       6 /            \ 6
       4 /   Pushups   \ 4
       2 /  and Dips    \ 2
```

```
              20
          27 /\ 27
         24 /    \ 24
        21 /      \ 21
        18 /      \ 18
       15 /        \ 15
       12 /        \ 12
        9 /          \ 9
        6 /           \ 6
        3 /   Situps    \ 3
```

Total: 200 pushups
300 situps

8-Count Body Builders 20

Platoon Run 2 miles

97

WEEK # 3 NO RUNNING

MONDAY	TUESDAY	WEDNESDAY
UPPER BODY PT	LOWER BODY PT	UPPER BODY PT

MONDAY

UPPER BODY PT

Warmup: 1/4 mile jog

Stretch: 10 min.

Two Sets of:

Pushups	20
Situps	30
Wide Pushups	20
Crunches	40
Triceps Pushups	15
Regular Crunches	50
8-Count Body Builders	10
Reverse Crunches	50
Dive Bombers	15
Left Crunches	50
Right Crunches	50
Arm Haulers	50

Stretch LEGS well!!
Especially Shins /
Achilles / ITB / Ham-
strings

TUESDAY

LOWER BODY PT

Warmup: 1/4 mile jog

Stretch: 10 min.

Legs	Reps
Squats	3 x 20
Lunges	3 x 20
Calf Raises	3 x 25
Sprints	2 x 50m
	2 x 75m
	2 x 100m
Dirty Dogs	3 x 40

Abs Super Set

Timed Curl-ups	
40 in 1 min. x 2	
30 in 45 sec. x 2	
20 in 30 sec.	
Crunches	4 x 40
Leg Levers	25
Flutter Kicks	100

WEDNESDAY

UPPER BODY PT

Warmup: 1/4 mile jog

Stretch: 10 min.

Pushups	Reps
Regular	4 x 25
Triceps	4 x 15
Wide	4 x 20
Dive Bomber	20
8-Count	20
Arm Haulers	50
L/R Side Crunches	50

WEEK # 3

THURSDAY

FRIDAY

SATURDAY

THURSDAY	FRIDAY	SATURDAY
TAKE A DAY OFF AND REST!	UPPER BODY PT	LOWER BODY PT

FRIDAY — Upper Body PT

Warmup: 1/4 mile jog

Stretch: 10 min.

Pushups	Reps
Regular	4 x 25
Triceps	4 x 15
Dive Bomber	3 x 10
8-Count	2 x 15
Arm Haulers	2 x 40

Abdominals

Curl-ups	50 x 2
Crunches	20 x 2
Flutter Kicks	25 x 2
Leg Levers	25 x 2

SATURDAY — Lower Body PT

Warmup: 1/4 mile jog

Stretch: 10 min.

Legs	Reps
Squats	3 x 20
Lunges	3 x 20
Calf Raises	3 x 25
Sprints	2 x 50m
	2 x 75m
	2 x 100m
Dirty Dogs	3 x 40

Abs Super Set

Timed Curl-ups	40 in 1 min. x 2
	30 in 45 sec. x 2
	20 in 30 sec.
Crunches	4 x 40
Leg Levers	25
Flutter Kicks	100

Platoon Run
2 miles

Words of encouragement:

"This ship is built to fight. You had better know how."

—*Admiral Arleigh Burke*

WEEK # 4

MONDAY	TUESDAY	WEDNESDAY
UPPER BODY PT	LOWER BODY PT	UPPER BODY PT

MONDAY		TUESDAY		WEDNESDAY	
Warmup: 1/4 mile jog		**Warmup:** 1/4 mile jog		**Warmup:** 1/4 mile jog	
Stretch: 10 min.		**Stretch:** 10 min.		**Stretch:** 10 min.	
Pushups	**Reps**	**Legs**	**Reps**	**Repeat 10 times:**	
Regular	4 x 25	Squats	4 x 20	Jumping Jacks	10
Triceps	4 x 15	Lunges	4 x 20	Regular Pushups	10
Dive Bomber	3 x 10	Calf Raises	4 x 25	Arm Haulers	20
8-Count	2 x 15	Sprints	3 x 50m	1/2 Situps	20
Arm Haulers	2 x 40		3 x 75m		
			3 x 100m		
Abdominals		Dirty Dogs	3 x 50		
Timed Curl-ups		Flutter Kicks	100		
	40 in 1 min. x 2	Leg Levers	100		
	30 in 45 sec. x 2				
	20 in 30 sec.				
Crunches	4 x 40				
Leg Levers	25				
Flutter Kicks	100				
Platoon Run		**Platoon Run**		**Platoon Run**	
2.5 miles		2.5 miles		2.5 miles	

WEEK # 4

THURSDAY	FRIDAY	SATURDAY
TAKE A DAY OFF AND REST!	UPPER BODY PT	LOWER BODY PT

THURSDAY

TAKE A DAY OFF AND REST!

Words of encouragement:

"I will find a way or make one."
—Robert E. Peary

FRIDAY

UPPER BODY PT

10 Super Sets

Regular Pushups	10
Crunches	10
Wide Pushups	10
Situps	10
Triceps Pushups	8
Reverse Crunch	10

Complete each cycle 10 times within 2 minutes per cycle.

Total workout time: 20 minutes.

Platoon Run
2.5 miles

SATURDAY

LOWER BODY PT

Legs	Reps
Squats	4 x 20
Lunges	4 x 20
Calf Raises	4 x 25
Sprints	3 x 50m
	3 x 75m
	3 x 100m
Dirty Dogs	3 x 50

Platoon Run
2.5 miles

101

WEEK # 5

MONDAY	TUESDAY	WEDNESDAY
UPPER BODY PT	LOWER BODY PT	TAKE A DAY OFF AND REST!

MONDAY

UPPER BODY PT

Warmup: 1/4 mile jog

Stretch: 10 min.

Pushups	Reps
Regular	4 x 25
Triceps	4 x 15
Dive Bomber	3 x 10
8-Count	2 x 15
Arm Haulers	2 x 40

Abdominals

Timed Curl-ups
  60 in 1 min. 30 sec. x 2
  40 in 1 min.   x 2
  30 in 45 sec.   x 2
  20 in 30 sec.

Crunches	4 x 40
Leg Levers	25
Flutter Kicks	100

TUESDAY

LOWER BODY PT

Warmup: 1/4 mile jog

Stretch: 10 min.

5 Super Sets	
Squats	20
Situps	20
Lunges	20
1/2 Situps	20
Calf Raises	20
Crunches	20

Total Leg Exercises: 300
Total Abs: 300

Platoon Run
3 miles

WEDNESDAY

TAKE A DAY OFF AND REST!

Words of encouragement:

"Fight her 'til she sinks and don't give up the ship."
—*Captain James Lawrence of the U.S.S. Chesapeake, as he was carried below, mortally wounded, in his losing fight with the HMS Shannon.*

WEEK # 5

THURSDAY	FRIDAY	SATURDAY
LOWER BODY PT	UPPER BODY PT	LOWER BODY PT

THURSDAY — LOWER BODY PT

Warmup: 1/4 mile jog

Stretch: 10 min.

Legs	Reps
Squats	4 x 20
Lunges	4 x 20
Calf Raises	4 x 25
Sprints	4 x 50m
	4 x 75m
	4 x 100m
Dirty Dogs	100

Abdominals

Timed Curl-ups
60 in 1 min. 30 sec.	x 2
40 in 1 min.	x 2
30 in 45 sec.	x 2
20 in 30 sec.	x 2
Crunches	4 x 40
Leg Levers	25
Flutter Kicks	100

FRIDAY — UPPER BODY PT

Warmup: 1/4 mile jog

Stretch: 10 min.

15 Super Sets
Pushups	10
Crunches	10
Wide Pushups	10
Situps	10
Triceps Pushups	8
Reverse Crunch	10

Complete each cycle 15 times within 2 minutes per cycle.

Total workout time: 30 minutes.

SATURDAY — LOWER BODY PT

Warmup: 1/4 mile jog

Stretch: 10 min.

Legs	Reps
Squats	4 x 20
Lunges	4 x 20
Calf Raises	4 x 25
Sprints	3 x 50m
	3 x 75m
	3 x 100m
Dirty Dogs	100

Platoon Run

3.5 miles

103

WEEK # 6

MONDAY	TUESDAY	WEDNESDAY
UPPER BODY PT	LOWER BODY PT	TAKE A DAY OFF AND REST!

Warmup: 1/4 mile jog

Stretch: 10 min.

20 Super Sets

Pushups	10
Crunches	10
Wide Pushups	10
Situps	10
Triceps Pushups	8
Reverse Crunch	10

Complete each cycle 20 times within 2 minutes per cycle.
Total workout time: 40 minutes.

Platoon Run
3.5 miles

Warmup: 1/4 mile jog

Stretch: 10 min.

Legs	Reps
Squats	4 x 20
Lunges	4 x 20
Calf Raises	4 x 25
Sprints	3 x 50m
	3 x 75m
	3 x 100m
Dirty Dogs	100

Platoon Run
3 miles

Words of encouragement:

"I wish to have no connection with any ship that does not sail fast, for I intend to go in harm's way."
—*John Paul Jones*

WEEK # 6

THURSDAY	FRIDAY	SATURDAY
Lower Body PT	Upper Body PT	Take a day off and REST!

THURSDAY — Lower Body PT

Warmup: 1/4 mile jog

Stretch: 10 min.

Legs	Reps
Squats	4 x 20
Lunges	4 x 20
Calf Raises	4 x 25
Sprints	3 x 50m
	3 x 75m
	3 x 100m
Dirty Dogs	10

Abdominals

Timed Curl-ups	
80 in 2 min.	x 1
60 in 1 min. 30 sec.	x 2
40 in 1 min.	x 2
30 in 45 sec.	x 2
20 in 30 sec.	
Crunches	4 x 40
Leg Levers	25
Flutter Kicks	10

Platoon Run
3.5 miles

FRIDAY — Upper Body PT

Warmup: 1/4 mile jog

Stretch: 10 min.

Two Sets of:

Pushups	50
Situps	50
Wide Pushups	30
Crunches	50
Triceps Pushups	25
Regular Crunches	50
8-Count Pushups	20
Reverse Crunches	50
Dive Bombers	15
Left Crunches	50
Right Crunches	50
Arm Haulers	50
Flutter Kicks	50

SATURDAY — Take a day off and REST!

Parent's Weekend!!!!

Remember:

"My country! May she ever be right, but right or wrong, my country."

—*Stephen Decatur*

RESTING, WORKING, AND MAXIMUM HEART RATES

Heart rates are excellent indicators of cardiovascular fitness. It is important to understand aspects of resting, working, and maximum heart rates in order to determine if you are getting a good aerobic workout, or to measure the level of intensity of your workout. For example, by comparing your working heart rate to your required working heart rate, you will be able to determine if you're going fast enough in a running workout or exercising hard enough during PEP.

To take your pulse, place your index and middle fingers on your wrist pulse point. Your pulse can also be taken in a similar manner along the carotid artery on your neck.

Working Heart Rate (WHR). Your working heart rate is established during any chosen exercise of any nature. Stop during any point in your exercise routine and count your heart rate for 10 seconds. Multiply by 6 to establish your working heart rate.

Resting Heart Rate (RHR). Your resting heart rate is established when first awakening in the morning. Count your pulse for 60 seconds before rising. Do this on 3 different mornings and use the average of the counts. The higher the degree of fitness, the lower the resting heart rate. FYI: The average midshipmen's resting heart rate is 66 beats per minute.

Maximum Heart Rate (MHR). Your maximum heart rate is measured by pushing yourself to MAXIMUM capability in any endurance event, then stopping and instantly taking your heart rate for 10 seconds. For example, run 880 yards at maximum speed. At completion, count your pulse at the carotid for 10 seconds and multiply by 6. Another way to find your maximum heart rate is to subtract your age from 220. For example, if you are 25, your maximum heart rate will be 195 (220-25).

Finding your maximum heart rate is essential in testing the intensity of your workout. As you approach your maximum heart rate, a seasoned athlete is performing at a very challenging level, but a novice is working out too hard and needs to slow down. As well, as you near or surpass your maximum heart rate, your workout switches from aerobic (burning fat) to anaerobic (burning blood sugar). Your body can only burn so much blood sugar until you burn out; hence the reason why you can't sprint as far or as long as you can jog. Try working out at 65 to 85% of your maximum heart rate to optimize the potential of your workout.

Required Working Heart Rate (RWHR). To establish the required training rate for cardiovascular fitness, the following formula may be used. Subtract your resting heart rate from your maximum heart rate. Calculate 75% of the difference. To that result, add your resting heart rate.

Example. If a midshipman has the following heart rates (MHR = 200 beats/min; RHR = 60 beats/min), the required working heart rate would be calculated as follows: 200 - 60 = 140; 75% of 140 = 105; add 60 and the result is 165 beats/min. This is the number of beats required by this subject to achieve a training effect in cardiovascular fitness.

Formula: RWHR = .75 (MHR - RHR) + RHR

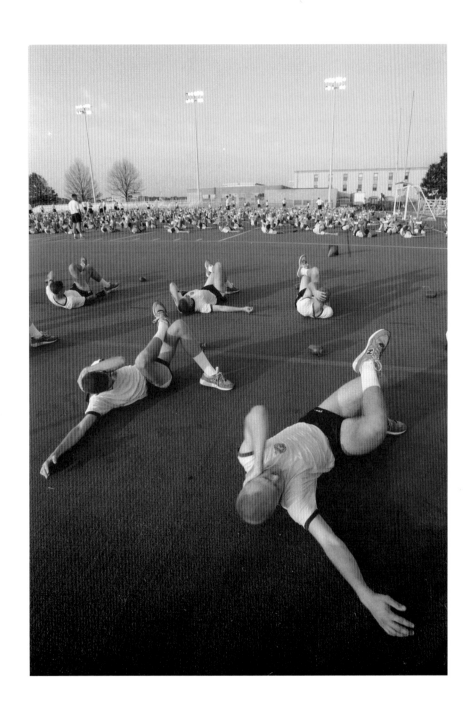

WORDS ON INJURY PREVENTION

There is no substitute for proper technique in avoiding injuries during your workouts. Many times people observe others exercising and attempt the exercise themselves without proper instruction. Needless to say, a good exercise performed incorrectly can cause potentially serious injury! Knees, shoulders, and the lower back are commonly subject to injury, and as such, care should be taken to learn and perform exercises properly.

In addition, lack of warmup and stretching before exercising, stretching too intensely or when you are not warmed up, and bouncing while you stretch are potential causes of physical injury.

The anchor is "aweigh" as soon as it is no longer touching the bottom.

Running is another common source of injury, and as a midshipman or recreational runner, it is important to take precaution to prevent injuries. Injuries often associated with running include stress fractures and shin splints. One of the best ways to prevent stress fractures is to stage your running program carefully. Intense running for several weeks makes your bones more susceptible to stress fractures, so taking time off from running is an important component. For more on developing a running program designed to minimize stress fractures, read Stewart Smith's *Complete Guide to Navy SEAL Fitness.*

Shin splints are a common and painful running injury. The shin is composed of the tibia and the fibula bone shafts. The tibia transmits the weight of the body to the foot. Lying between the tibia and the fibula are membranes which have a poor blood vessel system. Unless you warm up and exercise properly, the constant pull of the leg muscles against the connecting membranes frequently causes inflammation and irritation of the membranes. The result is pain. There is evidence that proper exercises contribute to the prevention of shin splints.

EXERCISES FOR PREVENTING SHIN SPLINTS

EXERCISE #1: Assume a deep squat position, with your soles and heels flat on the deck. Keep your hands in front on the deck for balancing. Move back and forth, side to side, rotating clockwise and counter-clockwise. Do this for 1 to 2 minutes.

EXERCISE #2: Done with a partner. Lie on your back. Your partner should grasp the toes of both of your feet. While on your back, pull your toes toward your knees. Hold that "stressed" position for 10 seconds. Repeat procedure 3 times. Switch positions and repeat accordingly.

Finally, it is important to get plenty of rest, eat right (see Words on Nutrition), and visit your doctor at least once a year for a proper check-up. If you follow careful, intelligent fitness protocol you'll have a safer, more productive workout and will spend less time in sick bay!

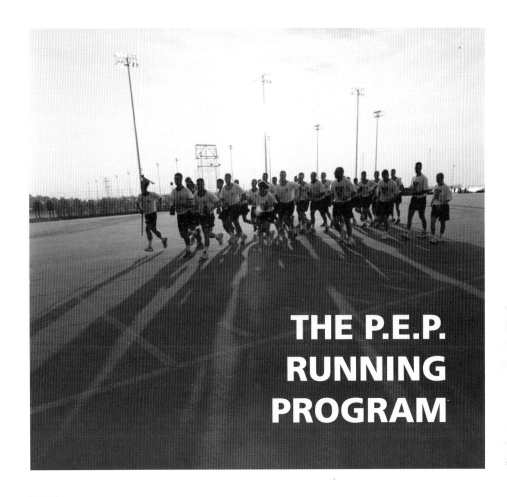

THE P.E.P. RUNNING PROGRAM

The P.E.P. running program is designed to prepare plebes to successfully complete the USNA PRT run.

For the first two weeks, all runs are platoon runs, concentrating on the development of platoon unity and spirit. The third week is a week of upper body and lower body PT only. There is no running during the third week. This is due to the high risk of stress fractures during the third week of any introductory exercise or running program.

The fourth, fifth, and sixth weeks allow all P.E.P. participants to compete against each other on Thursdays and Saturdays in a marathon-style run. Monday's platoon run remains the same throughout Plebe summer. The running goal by the end of the six-week program is:

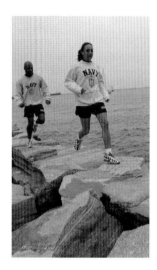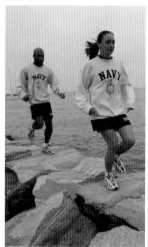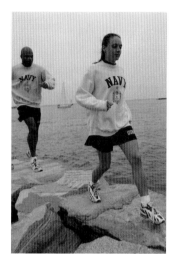

MEN:	7 min./mile minimum
WOMEN:	8 min./mile minimum

If a plebe fails to maintain the pace of the platoon this will result in he or she joining the "Motivation Squad." This group, led by a pre-designated officer or chief, conducts extra exercises such as sprints, lunges, grass-drills, and bear crawls in order to motivate the "slow" plebes to move a little faster.

RUNNING PROGRESSION CHART

WEEK 1:	1.5 miles
WEEK 2:	2 miles
WEEK 3:	NO RUNNING. High risk of stress fractures!
WEEK 4:	2 miles
WEEK 5:	3 miles
WEEK 6:	4 miles

THE SWIMMING PROGRAM

Midshipmen are required to be proficient in aquatics and to possess confidence in meeting emergency conditions in the water. This comes with the territory of being in the Navy and the likelihood of spending a significant portion of your career on a ship. If you aspire to be an Officer in the US Navy, many sailors will look to you for leadership in times of stress. History has demonstrated that comfort in the water and proper training in water survival techniques greatly reduces the chance of perishing at sea.

Hence, each Midshipman must demonstrate that he or she can swim and survive. Every year for the first three years, Mids are required to take a one hour class each week in swimming. They learn crawlstroke, breaststroke, sidestroke, backstroke, underwater swimming and water survival.

Here are the swimming requirements that each Midshipman must pass:

PLEBE YEAR
- 200m no greater than 5 min.12 sec.
- 5m tower jump
- 40' underwater swim

SOPHOMORE YEAR
- 400m no greater than 11 min.
- 10m tower jump
- 50' underwater swim

JUNIOR YEAR
- 40 minute swim in khaki pants and shirt
- 1000m in 40 min.

If a midshipman needs remedial training in swimming it is available 5 days a week.

Bottom line: Don't be an aqua-rock! Swimming is an excellent cardiovascular exercise. It works a majority of your major muscle groups. Proper instruction in swimming and water safety should be sought by every capable person. It is a real confidence builder.

As this guide does not intend to present instruction in swimming, we recommend you contact the American Red Cross or your local YMCA or YWCA to find out more about swimming and water safety programs in your area. And remember: never swim alone!

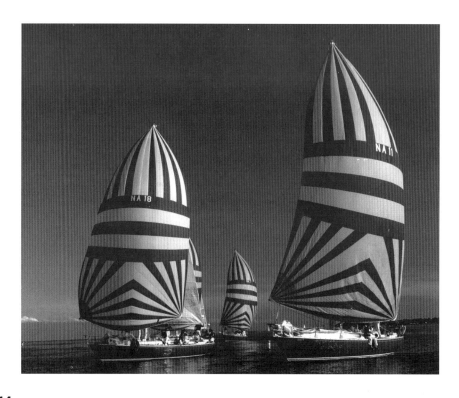

GLOSSARY

SELECTED NAVAL ACADEMY SLANG

AQUA ROCK: A non-swimmer; one in training for submarine duty but lacking a submarine.

BAGIT: Not attempting to perform to one's ability; taking the low road when everyone else takes the high road.

CAKE: Anything that is easy; dessert for which baggers have a recipe.

CHIT: Ticket for dining out and other privileges.

CHOP: To double-time; outdated plebe mass transit system.

CIVILIAN: A day with no classes.

CRABTOWN: Annapolis, a small village on the banks of the Naval Academy.

DECK: the floor (of the ship)

FIRST CLASS ALLEY: The walkways on the far sides of the Wardroom; place for the high and mighty to converse.

FORTY YEAR SWIM: Second class swimming marathon lasting forty continuous minutes.

GAS FACTOR: Inversely proportional to the happiness factor.

GUNGY: Psyched up for the Navy.

HAPPINESS FACTOR: The number of days of Christmas leave divided by the number of days until leave, an equation even the bull majors never forget.

HOP: Any Dance.

KAYDET: West Point Cadet; supplier of gray B-robes.

MIDDY: Midshipman; an odious term sometimes used synonymously with a Mid by mothers and newspapers.

MISERY HALL: First Aid rooms in MacDonough Hall and Halsey Field House; overhaul spot for damaged athletes.

MOTHER "B": Home of the Brigade, Bancroft Hall.

PLEBE: Fourth Classman; that insignificant thing that gets all the sympathy and chow from home.

PLEBE INFORMAL: Periodic mandatory Fourth Class mixers; just another Tea Fight.

PODUNK: Your home town.

RACK: Bed; the ultimate goal of most Midshipmen.

R.H.I.P.: Rank hath its privileges.

R.H.I.R.: Rank hath its responsibilities.

SECOND CLASS ALLEY: The spaces between the Wardroom tables; reward for a seven year commitment.

SIX-N DAY: Six classes in one day, i.e. no rack periods.

SMACK: Obsequious (and one who looks it up).

SNAKE: One who always has a date—someone else's.

STAR: To have a G.P.A. of 3.4, and A in conduct and performance, and at least a B in physical education.

STEERAGE: Cafeteria beneath Main-0; Center of Bancroft Hall night life.

SWEAT: One who worries excessively about everything. One who Brasso's his glasses. His room smells like Pledge.

UNREG: Unauthorized; not according to the Commandant.

WOOP: Kaydet; gray inmate of that isolated government institution which overlooks the Hudson.

YARD (THE): The United States Naval Academy.

Y.P.s: Yard Patrol Craft; corvette of the Fleet.

YOUNGSTER: Third Classman; plebes with carry-on stripes.

YOUNGSTER AFTERNOON: No 5th and 6th period in a day; sports period for Varsity Rack.

ZOOMIE: Air Force Cadet; one of our collegiate buddies who lives at the government play school in Colorado Springs and wears a blue bus driver cap.

ADMISSIONS CONTACT POINTS

For general information or a Precandidate Questionnaire, call the Candidate Guidance Office at
(410) 293-4361
Toll-free at:
1-800-638-9156, or write:

Candidate Guidance Office
United States Naval Academy
117 Decatur Road
Annapolis, MD 21402-5018

When writing to the Academy please be sure to include your full name and mailing address, including your zip code, year of high school graduation and if you would like your local Naval Academy Information Program Representative ("Blue and Gold Officer") to contact you. Please also include your phone number, including area code.

or visit the United States Naval Academy Website at
www.usna.navy.mil

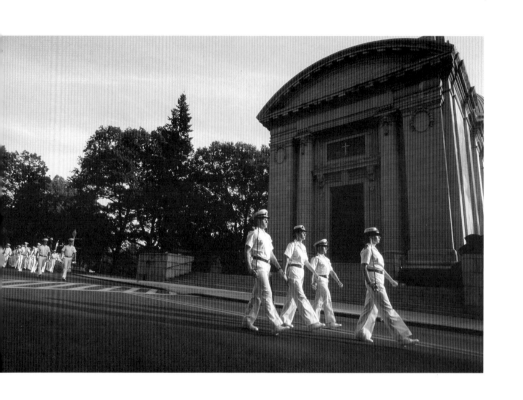

VISITORS INFORMATION

The Armel-Leftwich Visitor Center is open from 9 am to 5 pm, March through November, and from 9 am to 4 pm, December through February. Guided tours of the Academy are also available. Tours are available as follows:

June through Labor Day: Monday to Saturday, 9:30 am-3:30 pm, and Sunday 12:30-3:30 pm, every half hour.

September through November, and March through Memorial Day: Monday to Friday, 10 am-3 pm, hourly; Saturday, 10 am-3:30 pm, every half hour; and Sunday 12:30-3:30 pm, every half hour. *From Monday through Friday, noon tours will leave at 11:45 am to see the Noon Meal Formation.

December through February: Monday through Saturday, 11 am & 1 pm; Sunday, 12:30 pm & 2:30 pm.

For more information please call the Information & Guide Service at 410-263-6933

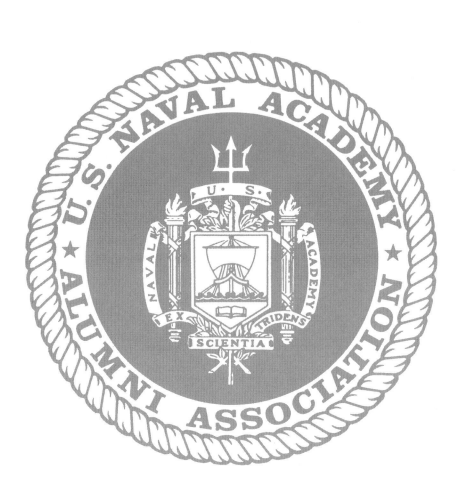

THE UNITED STATES NAVAL ACADEMY ALUMNI ASSOCIATION

We are pleased and proud to donate a portion of the proceeds from the sale of this book to The United States Naval Academy Alumni Association. The United States Naval Academy Alumni Association is a non-profit organization which plays a major role in supporting the Naval Academy through private gifts. In this capacity the Alumni Association provides a significant portion of the "value added" programs and opportunities at the Naval Academy.

THE ALUMNI ASSOCIATION MISSION

To serve and support the United States, the Naval Service and the Naval Academy:

• By furthering the highest standards at the Naval Academy;

• By seeking out, informing, encouraging and assisting outstanding, qualified young men and women to pursue careers as officers in the Navy and Marine Corps through the Naval Academy; and

- By initiating and sponsoring activites which will perpetuate the history, traditions, memories and growth of the Naval Academy and bind Alumni together in support of the highest ideals of command, citizenship and government.

FOR MORE INFORMATION, WRITE:

USNA Alumni Association
247 King George Street
Annapolis, MD 21402-5068

Or visit their website at
www.usna.com

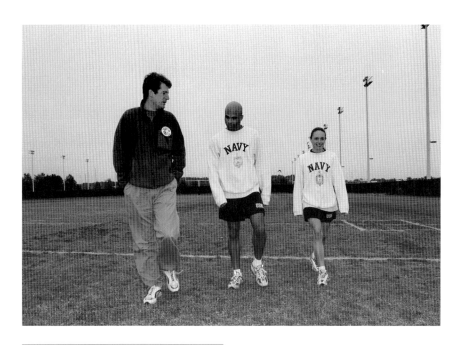

ABOUT THE AUTHORS

ANDREW FLACH

A lifelong fitness enthusiast, Andrew was born and raised in New York City, and is a graduate of St. David's School, The Browning School, and Vassar College. When he is not running a multi-million dollar media business, his recreational pursuits include sailing, mountaineering, rock climbing, mountain biking, SCUBA diving, and flying. He still resides in New York City.

PETER FIELD PECK

Peter Field Peck is a freelance photographer. His work has appeared in newspapers, magazines, and books. He currently resides in Brattleboro, Vermont.

The United States Marine Corps Workout

Researched by Andrew Flach
Photographed by Peter Field Peck

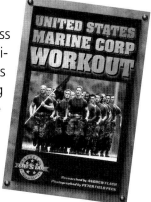

Witness the Leathernecks in action! For this fitness adventure, you'll join Charlie Company at the Officer's Candidate School at the US Marine Corps Base in Quantico, Virginia. You'll discover training techniques you've never seen before. These are rugged workouts for the rugged soul. You want to get fit? Tell it to the Marines!

You'll learn:

- Techniques to improve your upper body, lower body, and abdominal strength
- How the Marines prepare mentally for their grueling workouts
- Tips on running and endurance
- Traditions and customs of the Marines
- Total body workouts...plus dozens of powerful photos!

Whether you want to be a Marine or just be as tough as one, this is one book you don't want to miss. Semper Fi!

Just $14.95!
plus $3.00 S/H
ISBN 1-57826-011-6

To order call toll-free 1-800-906-1234

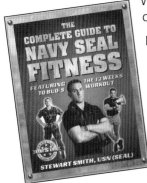